History, Science, and Politics

Influenza in America 1918–1976

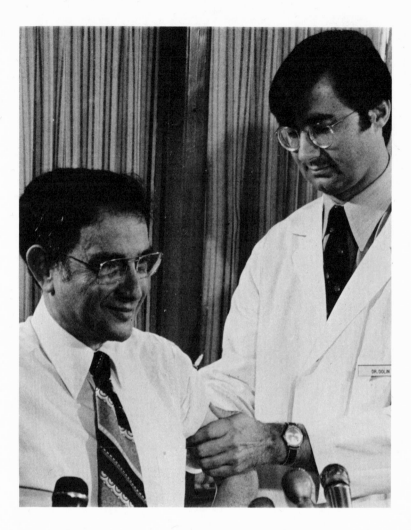

History, Science, and Politics

Influenza in America
1918 – 1976

JUNE E. OSBORN

Editor

1977

PRODIST

New York

PRODIST,
a division of
Neale Watson Academic Publications, Inc.
156 Fifth Avenue
New York, New York 10010

Library of Congress Cataloging in Publication Data

Main entry under title:

History, science, and politics.
Influenza in America 1918–1976
    Includes bibliographies.
    CONTENTS: Crosby, A.W., Jr. The pandemic of 1918.
—Millar, J.D. The scientific basis for the 1976
immunization campaign.—Viseltear, A.J. Immunization
and public policy.
    1. Influenza—United States—History. 2. Swine
influenza—United States—Preventive inoculation.
3. Influenza—United States—Preventive inoculation.
4. Medical policy—United States. I. Osborn,
June, 1937–   II. Crosby, Alfred W. The pandemic of
1918. 1977. III. Millar, John Donald, 1934–   The
scientific basis for the 1976 immunization campaign.
1977. IV. Viseltear, Arthur J. Immunization and
public policy. 1977.
RA644.I6H57   614.5'18'0973   77-14344
ISBN 0-88202-176-1

Designed and manufactured in the U.S.A.

Contents

Illustrations

Introduction

As a relatively influenza-free season drew to a close in the late winter of 1976–77, Professor Gunther Risse called me to discuss an idea. The fiftieth annual meeting of the American Association for the History of Medicine was to be held in Madison, Wisconsin, in May; and co-incidentally Professor Alfred Crosby had just completed a major study of the medical history of the 1918–1919 influenza pandemic. Dr. Risse knew of my involvement in the "swine flu" program and he therefore suggested enlisting Dr. Crosby as a speaker and asked my cooperation in preparing—and chairing—a symposium concerning the history, science and politics of influenza in America: 1918–1976.

Since I had been one of the government's embattled scientific advisors—in my case, to the Bureau of Biologics of the U.S. Food and Drug Administration—who had survived the previous year's events, the opportunity to bring all those perspectives to bear on the subject of pandemic influenza was most welcome and I agreed. While much had been written about A/New Jersey/76, alias "swine flu," a balanced view of the sort afforded by such a multifaceted approach had been hard to come by.

The symposium occurred, and the mix of disciplines was as exciting and effective as we had hoped, complete with insistent consumer groups eager to announce political "realities" which they perceived and feared we of the "establishment" might omit or whitewash. While not all the formal presentations at that symposium were in transcript and/or recorded form, this volume is specifically intended to recreate the effect of that meeting, with the salutory perspective created by a simultaneous analysis of the forces of history, science, and politics of twentieth century influenza which converged to create the "swine flu campaign of 1976."

Dr. Bruce Dull of the Center for Disease Control had been a most effective contributor to the symposium, delineating the scientific basis which had supported much of the initial decision-making in early 1976. Unfortunately, his talk was not recorded and as the decision to create this book was made he became ill, so

1

that Dr. J. Donald Millar and I cooperated to provide the necessary scientific details inherent in—but not always dominating—the ultimate political/economic decisions. The other two sections of the book—Dr. Crosby's and Dr. Viseltear's chapters—are essentially as they presented them at the Association's meeting.

This, then, is our plan. First, Dr. Crosby's contribution is a factual, startling evocation of the magnitude of the 1918–1919 pandemic. Raw mortality statistics tend to have a numbing effect rather than serving to alert or to alarm; and yet his focus on specific groups of people and, in particular, on the fate of the city of San Francisco and its citizenry serves to make real the appalling numerical toll of the great pandemic which killed half a million people in the United States alone.

With the scene thus set, Dr. Millar and I have tried in the second chapter to provide the background and vocabulary of scientific and biomedical considerations that led to the decision to embark on a national immunization campaign against the new strain of influenza virus that appeared early in 1976, properly designated as A/76/New Jersey. Some scientists might fault us for juxtaposing such a chapter with one about the 1918 virus, for when the new influenza strain appeared, careful scientists tried painstakingly to avoid the "scare" tactic of analogy to 1918. Nevertheless the similarity in antigenic properties was there and as they faced the possible reappearance of that deadly strain, shadows of memories pursued the older members of the biomedical community, while the under-55 group remembered fragments of lectures about the uniqueness and ferocity of the Great Pandemic. Both groups knew that despite the advances of medical science and public health practices, subsequent pandemics had been met with too little vaccine, too late.

Thus the apparent relatedness of the new strain to the 1918 influenza virus unquestionably helped to intensify concern among biomedical scientists, and the unusually good opportunity to take advantage of an adequate lead time in which to prepare vaccine before the next influenza "season" clearly helped to accelerate scientific decision-making. Peripheral considerations notwithstanding, however, those decisions were made carefully, scientifically, publicly and with all good intent by the several dozen highly trained advisors to the government.

In light of such conscientious good intentions Dr. Viseltear's contribution—a political history of the legislation that put the program into motion—is especially fascinating, since it inexorably leads from the initial painstaking analysis of benefits and risks, through the halls of Congress and into the glare of the Fourth Estate, to a legislative and administrative finale that has subsequently been called a "fiasco," a "disaster," a "debacle" and virtually any other florid descriptor available for use in situations where *post facto* vituperation becomes fashionable.

In the wake of that legislation, the public campaigns that followed, and the tribulations of the program, much occurred that undoubtedly will have far-reaching effects on subsequent programs in preventive medicine and public health. In an epilogue I have tried to add a brief history of those subsequent events along with my subjective view of the intangible costs and benefits resulting from the whole unprecedented experience.

I would like to acknowledge the able and rapid cooperation of the contributors to this volume, the initial sponsorship of the American Association for the History of Medicine, and most particularly the energy and enthusiasm of Dr. Gunther Risse, Professor and Chairman of the Department of the History of Medicine at the University of Wisconsin-Madison, whose initial inspiration sparked the symposium from which this volume derives.

June E. Osborn

INFLUENZA

FREQUENTLY COMPLICATED WITH

PNEUMONIA

IS PREVALENT AT THIS TIME THROUGHOUT AMERICA.

THIS THEATRE IS CO-OPERATING WITH THE DEPARTMENT OF HEALTH.

YOU MUST DO THE SAME

IF YOU HAVE A COLD AND ARE COUGHING AND SNEEZING. DO NOT ENTER THIS THEATRE

GO HOME AND GO TO BED UNTIL YOU ARE WELL

Coughing, Sneezing or Spitting Will Not Be Permitted In The Theatre. In case you must cough or Sneeze, do so in your own hand-kerchief, and if the Coughing or Sneezing Persists Leave The Theatre At Once.

This Theatre has agreed to co-operate with the Department Of Health in disseminating the truth about Influenza, and thus serve a great educational purpose.

HELP US TO KEEP CHICAGO THE HEALTHIEST CITY IN THE WORLD

JOHN DILL ROBERTSON
COMMISSIONER OF HEALTH

The Influenza Pandemic
of 1918

ALFRED W. CROSBY, JR.

The only specific event in history that compares with the world
wars of this century as a reaper of human lives is the influenza
pandemic of 1918–19. Like the world wars, the pandemic killed
tens of millions of people, but it was vastly more efficient: it did so
in less than a year whereas the wars took four or five years to
accumulate the same toll. The "Spanish Flu," as it was nick-
named in 1918, killed even more rapidly than the deadliest wars,
but not because it was as lethal to the individual sufferers as
bullets or bombs or plague or yellow fever. In fact, it rarely
dispatched more than two or three percent of its sufferers; but it
spread more rapidly and widely than any danger to human life
ever had before. By conservative estimate, a fifth of the human
race endured the fever and aches of influenza in 1918 and 1919,
and serologic evidence indicates that an enormous majority of
those fortunates who did not suffer the discomforts of flu did,
however, have subclinical cases of the infection. Having the
malady known as Spanish Flu was almost as characteristically
human at the end of World War I as having the opposable thumb.

Like the wars, this particular brand of influenza was, for
reasons that have never been satisfactorily explained, especially
dangerous to young adults. Although influenza did not significantly affect mortality in the United States until September, 1918,
its impact was so tremendous during the months that followed
that it wrenched the distribution of flu deaths by age of victim for
the entire year into unprecedented proportions (see Fig. 1). Since
the U.S. National Office of Vital Statistics started publishing data
on the age incidence of flu deaths, the distribution has been (as it
was in 1917, for instance) high at the extremes of infancy and old
age and very low in between; but in 1918 it was high for the very
young, higher yet for persons between twenty and forty, and

5

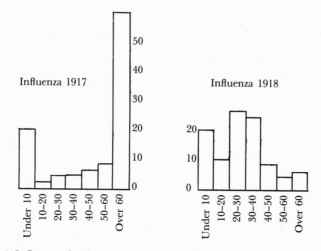

Fig. 1. Influenza deaths; percentage in each age group, U.S. Registration area, 1917, 1918 (after Jordan, Edwin, *Epidemic Influenza*).

lower than normal for the elderly. Thus the Spanish Flu had two outstanding characteristics: it killed millions of people, and most of them were in the prime years of life.

This distinctive influenza swept over humanity in three major waves in 1918 and 1919. We cannot be sure where the first wave in the spring of 1918 originated, but the earliest scientific and statistical evidence of its world debut appeared in the United States in March. It attracted very little attention because pneumonic complications were few and deaths fewer; it seemed no more than another bout with the kind of respiratory disease that so often circulates at that time of year. Only later, after the second and killer wave had drawn attention to any and all respiratory diseases of 1918, did the statisticians notice that an unusually large proportion of the few flu and pneumonia victims of the spring who died had been young adults.

This March and April wave expanded across North America, temporarily disrupting the operation of some military camps and a few factories, and then disappeared from the United States and Canada. As the flu waned in North America, it rose in the Old

World to greater heights than had been experienced since the last
pandemic of influenza in 1889–1890. According to the record (by
no means as complete in 1918 as today), the disease first reached
epidemic stage in Europe in the month of April in France. It
swept across the Continent in the spring and summer, sapping
the trench dwellers' devotion to battle (General Eric von Lüden-
dorff blamed the flu, among other factors, for halting Germany's
last victory drive in July). The number of peaceful Europeans laid
low by the flu in the summer was equally impressive: 53,000 in
July alone in tiny Switzerland and so spectacularly many in
Spain that the world decided to call this new malady the Spanish
Flu.

The new flu showed up in North Africa in May, in Bombay
and Calcutta in June, and by the end of July half of Chungking
was sick with it. By then it had already reached New Zealand, the
Philippines, and Hawaii. Even in an age before air travel, influenza had circled the globe in less than five months.

But the pandemic still seemed no more dangerous than
previous such experiences: multitudes of people ill, offices, factories and, in that year, armies and navies occasionally disrupted,
but only a few stricken for more than a week and very few dying.
Of course, the number sick with flu was growing so enormous
that even the small percentage who contracted pneumonia and
died was becoming impressive; and, while some Jeremiahs were
pointing to the strangely large proportion of young adults among
the dead, on the whole the pandemic was still regarded as only a
hindrance and a distraction.

At the end of the summer of 1918, the world health picture as
viewed from America was encouraging although a little perplex-
ing. A pandemic of a new strain of flu had rolled over humanity
but was on the decline in August for apparent lack of fresh
populations to infect. Oddly, the United States where the new
strain may have originated had almost no influenza at all, although Americans were in daily contact via steamer with islands
and continents where the pandemic was then raging much more
fiercely than it had in American in the spring. The outlook,
however, seemed rosy.

The most apparent threat that influenza portended was that

the war had produced optimum conditions for the development of new variants of influenza viruses. Millions of people of the ages most susceptible to severe influenzal infection were jammed together in industrial cities, military camps and ships, and were shifting about the world in immense numbers. Americans were moving at a rate of two or three hundred thousand a month from influenza-free America to a Europe rife with the disease, which proffered a specially fertile opportunity to whatever forces control the development of new strains of microorganisms.

In late August the influenza virus changed suddenly into the most dangerous strain (or strains) of that organism of which we have any record. It did so in three major ports of the North Atlantic almost simultaneously: Freetown, Sierra Leone, where local West Africans mixed with British, South African, East African, and Australian soldiers and sailors and soldiers bound to and from the war in Europe; Brest, France, which was the chief disembarkation port for Allied troops; and Boston, Massachusetts, one of America's chief embarkation ports and crossroads for military and civilian personnel of every nation involved directly or indirectly with the Allied war effort. Within days thousands were sick and hundreds dying as the new strain or strains moved outward from these three foci.

From the end of August on, the record of the second wave of the 1918 flu had as many stories as there were nations, cities, villages, families and individuals stricken by the newly virulent disease. Three percent of the native population of Sierre Leone died in September. The new wave peaked in Boston and Bombay in the first week of October. The mortality in India that month, according to an official report, was "without parallel in the history of disease." In Western Samoa the disease struck an isolated and immunologically almost defenseless people in November and killed 7,500 of a total population of 38,000 in less than two months. Scores of thousands of soldiers on both sides of the Western Front were stricken, and the American Expeditionary Force's only full scale drive of the war—the Meuse-Argonne Offensive—sputtered and stalled as 69,000 medical cases, most of them flu and its complications, swamped an evacuation and hospital system already overtaxed with 93,000 wounded and gassed.

The German Revolution and the establishment of the German Republic stalled as the Prime Minister, Prince Max of Baden, groaned through his own case of flu. Seemingly all of the important figures of the era had, were having, or were about to have a bout with the Spanish Flu or at least some kind of respiratory illness that fall and winter: Prince Max, Lloyd George, Clemenceau, Colonel House, and Woodrow Wilson were all significantly ill, and the peace conference was nearly twisted into an even more appalling snarl than it was in already when Woodrow Wilson came close to death from influenza in April, 1919, at the tag end of the pandemic's third wave.

The full history of the pandemic cannot be encompassed by the human mind, so let us examine the experience of one city, San Francisco. The spring wave of the 1918 flu passed over the city, smothered a few victims in their sick beds, and broke without having stirred general or professional interest. The second wave could never have been so benign and retiring, no matter what the precautions, but it might have been less lethal than it proved to be if the warnings had been heeded. The staggering news of the September morbidity and mortality rates in Boston reached the West Coast several weeks before the full brunt of the pandemic, but the skepticism and confusion of officialdom and the simple ignorance of the general populace stalled preparations for its arrival. As the pandemic moved westward, nearly all American cities including San Francisco were concentrating on the marches and other public gatherings of the Fourth Liberty Loan Drive, activities which were virtually guaranteed to speed the spread of any and all communicable diseases. When the first case of the new flu (a traveller from Chicago) arrived on approximately September 23, barely a month after the first cases in Boston, Brest, and Freetown, the city of the Golden Gate was just beginning to focus its attention on the threat to its well-being.

Full preparations—the divisions of the city into districts, each with its own medical personnel, telephones, transportation and supplies; the creation of emergency hospitals in schools and churches; the recruiting of hundreds of drivers and other volunteers, etc.—were not completed until November, by which time the worst of the flu in San Francisco had abated. Should the city's leaders be condemned because they moved too slowly? Of course, but the situation was unprecedented, a little incomprehensible even to health professionals, and public apathy made any inconvenience to large numbers of people impossible. Our own adventures with "swine flu" in 1976 should persuade us to regard the unfortunate authorities of 1918 with sour sympathy rather than self-righteousness.

Moreover, the factor that overruled all others during the pandemic was not proper planning or the lack of it, but rather the velocity and magnitude of the shock wave of disease racing around the world. Take for example the story of the San Francisco Hospital, widely rated as the finest in the state with the best trained and disciplined staff. Its reputation earned it the privilege of being chosen as the city's isolation ward for cases of pneumonia during the pandemic, and it came within a hair of failing disasterously at the job. Seventy-eight percent of its nurses fell ill, and it is likely, considering the devotion to duty characteristic of the staff, that many of the "healthy" nurses should have gone to bed as well.

At the end of October the San Francisco Hospital had 1,100 patients packed under its roof whose pneumonias had nearly all been sparked by the flu, and the superintendent announced that there was not room in the wards, halls, or porches for so much as one more patient. Providentially the number of new flu and pneumonia sufferers began to drop precisely at that time and the hospital, teetering on the edge of chaos, did not quite go over. A few more days like those at the end of October and one of the finest hospitals in the nation would have collapsed, as did many of its second and third rate counterparts. During the pandemic the San Francisco Hospital admitted 3,509 cases of respiratory disease, of whom twenty-six percent died.

During October the city tried every technique, procedure, and remedy that had been used on the East Coast to cure or slow the advance of the Spanish Flu. Literature on how to avoid and/or survive influenza and its jackal, pneumonia, was widely distributed. All schools and places of public entertainment were closed. Thousands of citizens were inoculated with totally useless and possibly dangerous anti-flu vaccines imported from the East or whipped up like Grandma's applesauce cake on the spot (with due respect to Grandma, it should be commented that she was probably more careful about her recipes than were the exhausted and harassed bacteriologists and laboratory technicians of 1918).

Like several other western cities, San Francisco spent much of its anti-flu effort in producing gauze masks and persuading its populace to wear them. The city Board of Supervisors passed a law making the wearing of masks obligatory in all public places, and on October 22 the Mayor, the Board of Health, the Red Cross and other organizations exhorted in the San Francisco Chronicle: "WEAR A MASK and Save Your Life!" A mask was "99% Proof against Influenza."

For the next month the great majority of San Franciscans obeyed, and hundreds who did not paid fines and went to jail. On Armistice Day wildly enthusiastic crowds swirled up and down Market Street and spilled over into the rest of the city, and every ecstatic celebrant was surrealistically swathed in a white mask. Happily, the masks seemed to work. So did the vaccines and, in fact, so did all the other amulets that San Franciscans were clutching to shield themselves from sickness and death. In November, for reasons of its own, the flu slackened and the numbers of new cases dramatically declined.

On November 21 every siren in the city shrieked the message that the moment for unveiling had come, and the masks came off amid general scenes of hilarity and triumph. As of that day the total of flu cases and deaths in San Francisco was far below what had been predicted on the basis of experience in the eastern cities. Authorities and the general public credited the city's success to the mask.

It had been characteristic of communities on the East Coast to suffer one terrific wave of Spanish Flu and only ripples thereafter. In the West, in contrast, communities often had two major waves. Barely two weeks after San Franciscans took off their masks and preened themselves on "how gallantly the city of St. Francis behaved when the black wings of war-bred pestilence hovered over the city," the number of new flu cases began to ease upward. The chief of the Board of Health expressed the hope that they were mostly misdiagnosed colds, but soon an avalanche of new cases—5,000 in December alone—confirmed his fear that all that he and his colleagues had claimed had been premature: the Spanish Flu was back for another round.

The third wave, in San Francisco as elsewhere in the world, was less virulent and deadly than the second. It sent hordes more to their sick beds and a considerable number of them to their graves before finally abating in the spring of 1919, but the death rate per thousand of population was only half that of the peak week of round two. (It should be noted that some consider the influenza epidemic of 1920, which gave the United States its third worst flu year in this century, to be the fourth wave of the pandemic.)

The most memorable features of round three in San Francisco were what one normally expects of an anticlimax: foolish antics on the part of the protagonists. Medical authorities trotted out their vaccines again, but this time the audience showed little interest. The city government again made masks compulsory, but this time against the stiff opposition of Christian Scientists, civil libertarians, merchants worried about what masks would do to Christmas shopping, and people who were simply fed up with masks, flu, and everything else. One of the latter sent the chief of the Board of Health a bomb which didn't go off.

The most effective opponents to the masks were experts in the state and city public health departments. They pointed out that there seemed to be no consistent difference in morbidity and mortality between communities which had adopted the mask and those which had not. The San Francisco police complained that the ubiquity of masks were encouraging robbery. The San Franciscan politicians noted, as one Supervisor put it, that ninety-nine and one half percent of the city's citizens opposed the compulsory mask law. On February 1, 1919, the masks came off officially. They had in fact come off some days before.

San Francisco, a city of 550,000, had made widespread use of all known preventatives and remedies for influenza and pneumonia and had enforced ordinances for the control of the pandemic as stringent as any implemented in any of the larger cities of the United States; but unknown scores of thousands of her citizens had nevertheless fallen ill and 3,500 had died. The city's record was not very different from that of Boston, the first city to be struck without warning by the fall wave in America. In San Francisco, as elsewhere, nearly two thirds of those who died of flu and pneumonia were between ages twenty and forty.

By mid-spring of 1919, the third wave of the pandemic was over everywhere except in the remotest reaches of places such as Alaska and Melanesia. The virus of Spanish Flu declined in virulence in the 1920s and ceased to circulate among human beings by the end of the decade. Serological evidence suggests that it has been holed up ever since in the pigs of the Middle West and other areas of heavy swine population. It was a sword that hung over the head of Damocles; the decline in the tone of civilization since his time has been such that it is not a sword but perhaps a pig that hangs over ours.

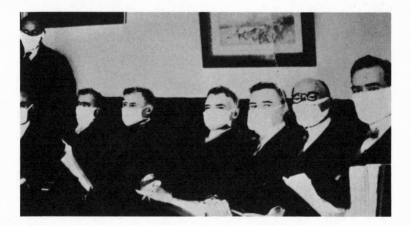

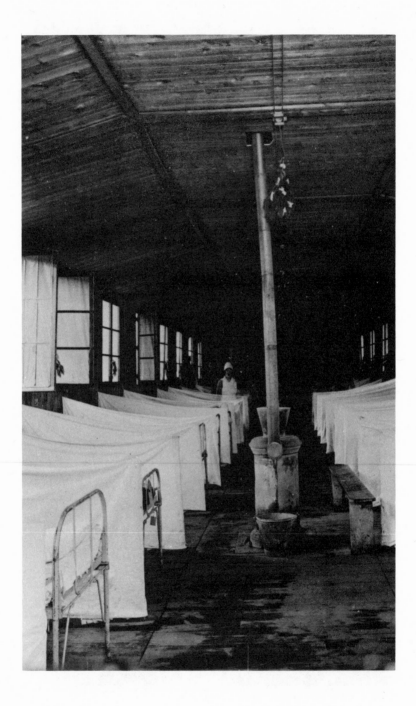

Precursors of the Scientific Decision-Making Process Leading to the 1976 National Immunization Campaign

J. DONALD MILLAR

AND JUNE E. OSBORN

The Great Pandemic of 1918–1919 occurred at a time when microbiology was an infant science. The germ theory of disease was generally accepted, some bacteria had complied sufficiently with Koch's postulates to be acknowledged as the cause of common diseases, and it was becoming evident that much smaller microorganisms—called viruses—sometimes played an equally virulent role in human contagious disease.[1] However, viruses were not yet cultivable and in fact, by definition, were too small to be seen with microscopes or retained by filters that readily held back larger microorganisms. Because of the rudimentary state of the art, therefore, the virus that caused the 1918–1919 pandemic was never captured. Later, when the technology for viral isolation had been developed, the desire to retrieve and study the killer strain was so strong that Alaskan flu victims were exhumed decades after their deaths in hopes that the culprit virus might have survived—but to no avail.

As a result we have only indirect clues to the nature of the pandemic influenza virus strain. Each influenza A virus has several distinctive antigenic proteins, and the mix of antibodies that an individual produces in response to those antigens is quite characteristic of a given strain. The antigenic "fingerprints" of the virus that caused the 1918–1919 disaster have been traced primarily by retrospective analysis of antibody patterns in the

15

blood serums of survivors. A person's first bout with an influenza
A strain tends to be the most immunologically memorable—that
is, subsequent infection with other (different) influenza A strains
induces not only new antibody patterns but also a return of
antibodies characteristic of the original viral antigens as well.
This phenomenon has the practical result, for our purposes, of
helping to identify and time the appearance of flu strains that
were prevalent in various eras. By studying people of appropriate
ages, then, scientists surmised that the 1918–1919 virus had antigenic characteristics unknown prior to that era and found since
the late 1920s only in swine. It was hypothesized that the swine
influenza virus might be the progeny of the killer strain, having
lost its ability to spread from human to human but retaining its
antigenic characteristics. The hypothesis that such a change in
virulence could occur without change in antigens may sound
somewhat strained, but molecular virologists have still not identified the particular combination of influenza genes that conveys
virulence and the incendiary capacity for man-to-man spread,
even though each gene of the flu virus today can be isolated and
its specific genetic message for nucleic acid and protein products
decoded.

The years between 1918 and 1976 were golden years for
microbiology and preventive medicine. Whereas the only effective
vaccine of that earlier era was against smallpox (one can still
argue about the efficacy of rabies vaccine), scientists began to
acquire improved skills to cultivate bacteria, to systematically
alter their virulence, or to isolate and change their toxic products,
all with the purpose of creating vaccines. Safe and generally
effective preparations became available to prevent bacterial diseases such as whooping cough and tuberculosis, diphtheria and
tetanus, and often dramatic declines in incidence of those diseases
followed.

But virology was slower than bacteriology to emerge as a
science, even though the first empirically attenuated vaccines had
been against viral diseases such as smallpox and rabies. The brake
on progress resulted from the stringent obligatory parasitism of
viruses: They can not multiply unless they invade and preempt

the metabolic machinery of another "host's" living cells—in sharp contrast to most bacteria, which can rapidly reproduce their kind simply with the help of agar and other chemically defined growth media. The profound dependency of viruses on living cells was not fully appreciated for many years, but in 1930 it was found that influenza virus could be grown in embryonated hens' eggs.[2] Shortly thereafter the same approach was used successfully to cultivate the virus that causes yellow fever. More dramatically, when yellow fever virus was subjected to egg-to-egg passage, the progeny virions were depleted of their disease-producing potential, while still retaining their ability to multiply enough in humans to stimulate antibody production. Thus not only were crude tools at hand to study some viruses nearly fifty years ago, but early successes at vaccine development were sufficiently exciting to lend great momentum to the pursuit of vaccines for many other diseases.

Another major advance in the science of influenza occurred in the early 1940s when it was found that the optically invisible virus could be tracked indirectly by its specific clumping effect on red blood cells—a phenomenon called hemagglutination. Furthermore the proteins of the virus that caused visible agglutination were also major antigens, and so specific antibodies could block the effect when they were mixed with the virus before red blood cells were added. This pair of techniques allowed for the measurement of virus and antibody concentrations, and, because of the individuality of each protein antigen, virologists then had tools of sufficient precision to explain the unique behavior of influenza among human viral pathogens. While all the other viruses had apparently immutable antigenic characteristics, influenza A virus clearly had the capacity to change its "antigenic spots." Indeed, it seemed to do so at approximately ten-year intervals, resulting in the intermittent worldwide epidemics of influenza which so color the history of the human race.

Immunity to a given strain of influenza A was as durable for the survivor of infection as was his immunity to measles, but the appearance of a new antigenic variant suddenly rendered that immunity virtually useless. Obviously this unique property of influenza virus, plus the very short incubation period of the disease, presented extraordinary problems to the makers of vaccines, for each time a new flu appeared they had to start over in the tedious process of preparing an effective vaccine.

However, vaccine makers are hard to discourage, and as long as influenza A viruses could be grown to high concentrations in embryonated hens' eggs, the road to vaccine development was open. Efforts to create an attenuated vaccine with altered virulence for humans were plagued with either too much or too little success[3]—in the former case the virus failed to multiply at all and therefore did not include antibodies, whereas in the latter case the "attenuated" virus still made recipients sick. So virologists concentrated on producing a so-called "killed" or inactivated influenza vaccine. They achieved this by growing virus in eggs in such quantities that enough viral antigens could be delivered in one "shot" to stimulate an antibody response without the need for viral multiplication.

Initially this approach was only partially successful: It was tedious and difficult to adapt fresh isolates of influenza to grow well in eggs. Furthermore, killed influenza vaccines varied somewhat in potency and packed a fairly stiff wallop in the form of sore arms and brief fevers a day or so after their injection. Worse yet, the inoculations had to be repeated at yearly intervals to sustain antibody levels adequate for protection against the prevalent flu virus.

Much of the problem lay in the relative impurity of early influenza vaccines, which contained residual egg proteins as well as influenza viral antigens. When purification techniques in the 1960s made it possible to remove all but the desired viral antigens, much of the unpleasant "reactogenicity" disappeared. Nevertheless, some of the unwelcome side effects seemed to be inherent in the purified killed virus itself, which still caused discomfort when doses above a certain threshold concentration were injected.

Despite early problems, by the mid-1950s these methods of preparing influenza vaccines were potentially available for use in prevention or control of future pandemics. Before recounting the experiences that followed, however, it is interesting to call to mind several other trends in the public's perceptions and expectations regarding health and disease that had developed in the years since 1918.

First, by 1976 the conquest of infectious diseases had seemed so nearly complete that the American public had forgotten (or had never known) the scourges for which vaccine prevention was being offered. For instance, during the first half of the twentieth century urban America had been terrorized with the increasing frequency and severity of summertime polio epidemics. The dramatic cessation of these fearsome episodes which followed the use of, first, killed and then attenuated polio vaccines is a proud and familiar story to physicians over the age of 45. But the miracles of Salk and Sabin vaccines had so paled by the 1970s that, though ingestion of a sugar cube laced with virus was all that was needed for protection, half the children of some communities had never been taken by their parents to receive polio immunization. The fearful dog days of the 1940s and 1950s, when strong healthy limbs could suddenly be shriveled for life, were remembered by a diminishing number of Americans, both physicians and public alike; the new generation of young parents had grown up in a polio-free era with the result that they felt little innate motivation to take advantage of immunization programs for their offspring.

The successful practice of public health requires salesmanship of a high order. But the sale of polio vaccine to an unmotivated public was seriously complicated in the 1970s by a less than one-in-a-million chance that paralysis could follow polio immunization. Although the paralysis usually could not be traced to the polio vaccine, it was touted by some critics as an intolerable price to pay for prevention of an obscure or forgotten disease. The "hard-sell" approach to prevention of polio was further compromised when a judge ruled that it was the vaccine manufacturer's duty, under penalty of law, to see that no dose of polio vaccine should be administered until the recipient had been lucidly warned that paralysis might follow, however miniscule the probability of that happening. The pharmaceutical industry was also faced with the diminishing availability of monkey kidney cells which were necessary for the growth of polio vaccine virus in tissue culture, for, like other once-abundant commodities, monkeys were in increasingly short supply. Vaccine production in general had never been particularly profitable for the industry and the burgeoning monster of possible litigation was threatening to consume the last vestiges of a rationale for participation in the business of polio vaccines. It appeared, then, by the mid-1970s, as though the wherewithal for poliomyelitis prevention might disappear entirely in the near future. Similar depressing tales could be told about measles and other preventable diseases.

In short, the very success of immunization programs during the 1950s and 1960s had led to an ablation in public memory of the scourges for which the vaccines had been created.

But a second remarkable change of the twentieth century must be emphasized. The American public's expectation of the medical profession had undergone profound alterations in the decades since 1918. At the time of the Great Pandemic, physicians were virtually powerless to influence the course of infectious diseases. Pneumonia, as everyone realized, was a disease about which there was nothing to do except watch and pray. Antibiotics were unknown, vaccines for respiratory infections were nonexistent, and so the doctor's role during an influenza pandemic was that of a kindly sage whose purportedly great learning allowed him to prognosticate wisely, but who completely lacked therapeutic weapons with which to intervene effectively.

Ironically, the very success of medical science subsequently distorted the image of its practitioners; improved sanitation and nutrition (still much the most significant advances in overall health care) and the creation or discovery of antibiotics and vaccines at first awed the public but later made them as demanding as spoiled children. Once cures for some diseases were available, it seemed intolerable that others still could not be checked. The availability of antibiotics introduced a major distortion in public perception of infectious diseases: surely everything could be handled with a "shot" if only a physician so chose; and many conscientious practitioners who withheld penicillin when they suspected viral rather than bacterial infection were deserted by their patients for more pliant therapists. The instant relief hoped for from an antibiotic "shot," therefore, was avidly sought, but the total prevention afforded by a vaccine shot was a bit of gratis discomfort which required a hard sell.

These considerations serve as a crucial backdrop to the story of influenza immunization. When the rather impure killed influenza vaccines became available in the 1950s, the groups of biomedical scientists who advised the medical community about immunization practices were restrained in their recommendations. Because of the mild but annoying side effects, it was generally felt that flu vaccine should be recommended only for persons whose benefit from protection against influenzal disease outweighed the risk of temporary fever and local discomfort following the immunization itself.

While the vaccines increased in purity and potency, the consistent advice of federally sponsored expert groups (until 1976) was that influenza vaccine be reserved for persons at "high risk" from the disease or its complications—groups such as the elderly and the chronically ill for whom a bout with flu might prove to be one stress too many. Federal agencies were involved in flu vaccine manufacture only in a regulatory way: they helped identify and certify significant new influenza virus strains and conducted the mandated potency testing and quality control of influenza vaccines. There was no federal financial support for administration of those vaccines to the special groups for whom they were recommended, and how much vaccine was to be produced was decided by pharmaceutical manufacturers whose dominant concern was what the market would bear. Their assessment usually resulted in the production of about 20 million doses of influenza vaccine per year for commercial distribution.

The results of that free market policy were not encouraging to public health workers. Since 1973, for instance, the Annual Immunization Survey had shown that the proportion of "high risk" persons who actually received those vaccine doses was strikingly low. In 1975, for example, less than 20 percent of the group for whom the vaccine was recommended were actually immunized; much of the remaining vaccine had gone to large corporations which purchased flu vaccine in bulk and administered it to their young, healthy employees to reduce wintertime attrition due to flu. This aspect of public policy concerning influenza vaccine therefore demonstrated a serious deficit in the existing system, assuming the experts' recommendations were sound.

Another way of looking at influenza vaccine experience before 1976 was to assess its role in prior pandemics. During the previous twenty years the nation twice faced imminent influenza pandemics which seemed to call for decisive action. In both cases we found ourselves far too late with far too little.

In February 1957 a major variant of influenza A virus initiated an epidemic in China which spread inexorably westward. Though the recommendation and subsequent decision were made to prepare vaccine, the federal government disdained to actively support a mass vaccination campaign. Funds were appropriated for surveillance, investigation, and even planning for disaster relief, but there was no financial support for the initiation of a national vaccination campaign. The vaccine formula against the so-called Asian flu strain was finally approved in July 1957 and vaccine production began.

It is a fact of life, however, that mass production of killed influenza vaccine requires a lead time of approximately six months: embryonated eggs are required in great quantity, the new virus strain is usually quite balky at first in its adaptation to growth in avian rather than human cells, and extensive quality and safety checks must be brought to bear on the product. (Happily our present, highly regulated society will not tolerate the free-wheeling approach of 1918 that "whipped up vaccines like Grandma's applesauce cake.") Furthermore, the best of killed virus vaccines still must be injected into the vaccinee at least three weeks before it conveys protection against infection. Therein lay the "too little and too late." By mid-October of 1957, when the epidemic reached its peak, less than 30 million doses of influenza vaccine had been fully tested for release, and only 7 million persons had actually received the benefit of immunization. The dismal price of failure was 70,000 deaths which could be ascribed to the influenza epidemic—and a large store of unutilized vaccine which had been produced too late to be of use.

In July 1968 a new pandemic threat was recognized when another major antigenic shift in influenza virus was detected in Hong Kong. By August the new strain was made available to manufacturers for production of vaccine. Despite an all-out production effort, the first lots of vaccine were not released until mid-November, three weeks *after* the first community-wide influenza outbreak in California. The epidemic rapidly spread eastward, infecting every state by Christmas. At the peak of the epidemic, only 10 million doses of vaccine had been distributed and no more than 6 million individuals had been protected; again, a large store of unused vaccine remained after the epidemic had passed. As noted earlier, vaccine production and sale is a relatively unprofitable activity for the pharmaceutical manufacturers (compared, for instance, to drugs of almost any sort), and such massive "bad gambles" are quite memorable to the executives who participate in decisions concerning vaccine production in subsequent years.

Therefore, though the response to the Hong Kong flu in 1968 was more brisk than to Asian flu in 1957, it was equally impotent in affecting the outcome. The excess death figure for the 1968–1969 pandemic in the United States was 33,000. That total was lower than the Asian flu toll, probably because the Hong Kong strain had only a single surface antigenic shift from preexisting A strains, with the result that the epidemic may have been somewhat blunted by partial pre-existing immunity.

Following both epidemics, there were considerable public grumblings about why sufficient vaccine had not been available when it would have done some good.

Those recent pandemic experiences pale by comparison with the Great Pandemic described in the previous chapter, and yet they demonstrate how enormously costly influenza can be. In monetary terms, detailed cost estimates for the 1968 epidemic total over $3,000,000,000 for the United States. By contrast, the cost of the 1918–1919 pandemic was estimated to be the equivalent (in 1968 dollars) of over $100,000,000,000. Moreover the mortality tolls of both the 1957 and 1968 pandemics, although awesome, were relatively minor when contrasted with the 500,000 Americans who had died in 1918. However, these experiences emphasized in inescapable terms to the biomedical and public health communities the need for haste if vaccine were to be employed as a weapon of mass prophylaxis in the face of a possible new pandemic.

By 1976 virologists were beginning to wonder when the periodicity of influenza's antigenic shifts would bring forth the next pandemic challenge, so it was alarming but not totally unexpected when a major new variant of influenza A virus was discovered at Ft. Dix, New Jersey in February, 1976. This virus caused an outbreak affecting several hundred recruits. It resembled influenza strains previously found in swine (hence "swine flu") and demonstrated major differences in surface antigens when compared with previously circulating influenza A strains. Always in the past such major variants had been associated with the onset of pandemics. Only persons over 50 years of age in the population had antibodies reactive to the newly recovered agent, suggesting that no one had experienced a similar virus since the 1920s. The remainder of the population would apparently be completely vulnerable to infection with the new strain, if the virus were to retain or increase its ability to spread among humans.

As inferred earlier, the best available but incomplete knowledge of "swine influenza" strains suggested that they appeared as a cause of human illness in 1917, produced the epidemic of 1918–1919, caused scattered human cases for several years thereafter, and in the late 1920s disappeared from the human population to persist in swine. Though isolated human cases began to reappear in 1973 from swine-to-man transmission, the Ft. Dix outbreak was the first time since the 1920s in which human-to-human transmission was clearly documented. Those observations suggested that the new strain recovered at Ft. Dix (labeled A/New Jersey/76) possessed pandemic potential. A national decision in regard to these findings was clearly required. Procrastination had doomed any possibility of protecting the population in 1957. In 1968, while the decision to produce vaccine was reached rapidly, the epidemic was on our shores before the minimum time required for vaccine production had elapsed.

However, in 1976 the situation was more favorable. Although a potential pandemic strain had appeared, it was recovered late in the flu season. Fully six months were available before the beginning of the next flu season, six months in which to prepare, test, and then administer a specific protective vaccine on a mass basis. An unprecedented opportunity existed to prevent much death and destruction if rapid action were taken. (Vaccine against A/Victoria influenza, the prevalent strain of that winter, had already been made in bulk in anticipation of the usual commercial market for about 20,000,000 doses.)

The options were straightforward: the government could do nothing other than provide the manufacturers with the new A/New Jersey/76 strain for production as usual; they could stimulate large-scale production of A/New Jersey/76 vaccine but withhold its use, creating a stockpile which could, it was hoped, be mobilized if there were further evidence of spread of the virus; or they could not only stimulate large scale production but also participate in administering the vaccine to the entire population as quickly as it became available. The "do-nothing" option was rejected as being irresponsible; the "stockpile" option was also rejected as involving the same race with time that had ended in stark failure in 1957 and 1968. Thus the decision was reached by the federal government, after consultation with dozens of advisors, to make A/New Jersey/76 vaccine and to mount a mass vaccination campaign to protect the entire population of the United States as rapidly as possible.[4]

Strange things were later said about the way these decisions were reached. There were charges of a "closed process," of ultra-secrecy, or of stifled dissent. In general there was the strong inference by later critics that some kind of self-serving influence permeated the selection of expert advisors and their subsequent decisions. It is noteworthy, therefore, that the U.S. Public Health Service Advisory Committee on Immunization Practices, supplemented by the Food and Drug Administration's Advisory Panel on Viral and Rickettsial Vaccines, and large numbers of additional experts helped develop and concurred in the decision to implement mass vaccination. This decision was reviewed in three distinct public meetings, and in each instance the experts affirmed their support.

Subsequently the much publicized White House conference of over 50 respected leaders in and out of science was convened, heard the evidence of the man-to-man spread of the new strain at Ft. Dix, and publicly affirmed support for the decision to conduct universal mass vaccination.

Finally, as discussed in the following chapter, a national immunization plan was almost unanimously endorsed by Congress which authorized a $135,000,000 budget for its implementation. During this phase and later, one or another aspect of the program was examined and re-examined in no fewer than 10 subsequent congressional oversight hearings.

In none of these fora of mid-1976 was the consensus to conduct mass production of vaccine openly disputed. While the "stockpile" argument did simmer publicly between Drs. Sabin and Salk (the former contending that the actual delivery of vaccine should be deferred until the reappearance of "swine flu"), no major responsible voice was raised against the program of mass production per se. Those arguments came later; but in the calm of consensus in April of 1976 Dr. Theodore Cooper, then Assistant Secretary of Health in HEW, administered the first dose of "swine flu" vaccine to Dr. Harry M. Meyer, Jr., Director of the Bureau of Biologics of the FDA. All decisions had been made and the testing of the new vaccine was under way.

References

1. For a full treatment of the evolution of the concept of a "virus," see *The Virus: a history of the concept* by Sally Smith Hughes (New York, Science History Publications, 1977).

2. For a full treatment of the scientific history of influenza virus, see *Influenza: the Last Great Plague* by W.I.B. Beveridge (New York, PRODIST, 1977).

3. Live attenuated influenza vaccines have in fact been developed in recent years. They hold considerable promise for the future but are still in an experimental stage at this writing.

4. Because A/Victoria vaccine was available in bulk, a corollary decision was reached to combine that material with some of the A/New Jersey antigen in a bivalent product for administration to persons considered at high risk from influenza. As everyone needed vaccination against the new A/New Jersey strain, no need was seen for a monovalent A/Victoria vaccine.

Influenza viruses also come in a "B" variety for which a vaccine was commercially available, but since influenza B viruses are not as clearly associated with high mortality, the B antigens were not included in the vaccine for the national program.

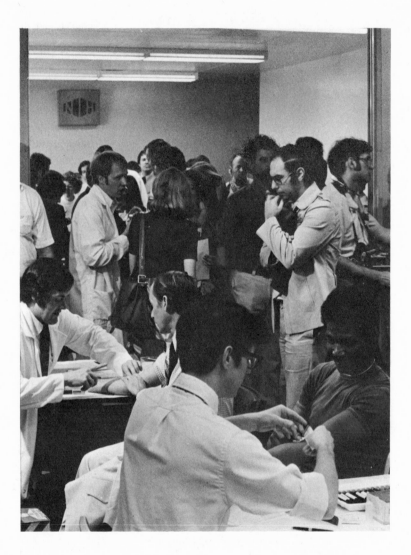

A Short Political History
of the
1976 Swine Influenza Legislation

ARTHUR J. VISELTEAR

"Sweet peace be his, who wipes the weeping eye,
And dries the tear of sobbing misery!
Still higher joys shall to his bosom flow,
Who saves the eye from tears, the heart from woe!
—A far, far greater honor he secures,
Who *stops the coming ill,* than he who cures."

—Valentine Seaman to Samuel Scofield,
letter dated August 15, 1809, in Samuel
Scofield, *A Practical Treatise on Vaccina
or Cowpock* (New York: Southwick and
Pelsue, 1810), p. v.

During the 94th Congress (1974–76), the health subcommittees in the House of Representatives and the Senate had a full agenda.[1] Authorizing legislation for a number of important health concerns was to expire, which would necessitate the revising and redrafting of existing legislation, the orchestration of hearings, the preparation of staff and member briefs, the scheduling of subcommittee and committee markups, floor debates and conferences, and the development of strategies and counterstrategies in preparation for the countless real and imagined threats and challenges which so easily frustrate legislative intent.

It would not be an easy Congress for the members and staffs of these committees, because of the tensions that perforce develop when the administration is of one party and the Congress of another, and also because of the sheer pressure of the legislative agenda, which included an omnibus and controversial medical manpower bill, amendments to the health maintenance and emergency medical services acts, a revised clinical laboratories improvement bill, and a comprehensive nurse training and health revenue package.

Nor would it be an easy Congress for other reasons as well— 1976, after all, was an election year. And it was also the Bicentennial. Congress and the nation would renew their collective faith in our country's historic mission and greatness, revel in past glories and, in speech after speech, extol the virtues of being an American while offering visions of the greatness of what might yet be. We had survived as a nation for over 200 years; there was nothing that could not be done if we but had a mind to do it.

Events occurring in Fort Dix in early 1976, however, were to test the pervasive optimism of our bicentennial rhetoric.

The facts were as follows:

1. In February 1976 a new strain of influenza virus was isolated.
2. The virus was determined to be antigenically related to the influenza virus which had been implicated as the cause of the 1918–1919 pandemic.
3. The entire U.S. population under the age of 50 was believed to be susceptible to this new strain.
4. Prior to 1930 this strain was the predominate cause of human influenza in the United States. Since 1930 the virus had been limited to transmissions among swine with only occasional transmission from swine to man—with no secondary person-to-person transmission.
5. In an average year, influenza causes about 17,000 deaths and costs the nation approximately $500 million; in pandemic years, such as 1968–1969, influenza struck 20 percent of our population, causing more than 33,000 deaths, and cost an estimated $3.2 billion.

These items were discussed by the Center for Disease Control's (CDC) Advisory Committee on Immunization Practices as soon as the virus' identity was confirmed.[2] The committee's basic concern was to determine how the federal government was to respond to the influenza problem caused by the new virus. After the lengthy debate Dr. David Sencer, CDC's director, prepared an "ACTION" memorandum,[3] which was to have the effect of mobilizing the vast resources of the Department of Health, Education, and Welfare (DHEW) and to shake this government's preventive health apparatus to its very core.

In the memorandum, which eventually found its way to the President, the basic assumption was that the evidence indicated that the "ingredients for a pandemic" were present. The situation called for a "go or no-go" decision for there was "barely enough time to assure adequate vaccine production and to mobilize the nation's health care delivery system." Therefore, the decision at hand had to be "immediate."[4]

Since there was no medical or epidemiological basis or rationale for excluding any part of the population, a second assumption was that the goal would be to immunize the total U.S. population. Owing to the fact that this nation had never attempted an immunization program of such scope and intensity, the federal government would have to provide leadership, sponsorship, and financial support.

The four courses of action set forth in the memo were for DHEW to take "no action," to "respond minimally," to develop a virtually "total governmental program," or to develop a consolidated or "combined effort" taking advantage of the strengths and resources of both the public and the private sectors. The alternatives covered every conceivable option, including politics, and some which the author of the memorandum doubtless considered intellectually and morally indefensible.

To take no action, owing to the fact that there was then only one frank case of swine flu, for example, would mean that the "market place" would prevail and that DHEW would have "avoided unnecessary health expenditures." Moreover, "direct federal intervention" was believed to be "contrary to current administration philosophy." On the other hand, the Congress, the media, and the American people would certainly expect the government to take some action. The administration, moreover, could tolerate unnecessary health expenditures far better than it could unnecessary death and illness. And, in all likelihood, Congress would certainly "act on its own initiative."[5]

The minimum response analysis envisioned a program whereby the federal government would be visible but would effect a partnership with the private sector and rely on existing delivery systems. It was a response predicated on minimum federal intervention and diffused liability and responsibility. Moreover, the burden on the federal budget would not exceed $40 million, considered a modest investment. The problem with this option was that there was little assurance that the vaccine manufacturers would undertake the massive production effort necessary. Under this option, therefore, less than half of the population were expected to receive their immunizations.[6]

If the federal government took over total responsibility for the program, the Public Health Service would then purchase the vaccine, and the state health departments would organize and implement the program. This alternative would assure universal distribution of the vaccine, would mean that economic status would have no bearing on accessibility, and would maintain traditional state and federal relationships for communicable disease control. Yet this third alternative would prove costly, approaching the $190 million level. Furthermore, it was believed to be "inefficient" to the extent that it failed "to take advantages of the private sector health delivery system," placed too much reliance on public clinics and government action, and was "contrary to the spirit and custom of health care delivery in this country."[7]

The final option would have relied on the federal government for its leadership, coordination, and purchasing power; on state agencies for their experience in conducting immunization programs and as logical distribution centers for vaccine; and on the private sector for its medical resources.

The concluding sentence of this fourth option indicated what CDC's recommendation would be. It read as follows: "Undertaking the program in this manner would provide a practical contemporary example of government, industry, and private citizens cooperating to serve a common cause—an ideal way to celebrate the nation's 200th birthday."[8]

The memorandum, dated March 13, 1976, made its way upward to the Assistant Secretary for Health who forwarded it to DHEW's Secretary David Matthews, a non-physician who was formerly President of the University of Alabama. It was then sent, virtually unchanged, to the Office of Management and Budget, the Domestic Council, and finally to the President.

The ultimate recommendation to the President was to accept CDC's conclusions that the combined federal-private program be implemented, but first to bring together a panel of experts to add additional authority to the final decision of the President. On March 24, such a panel was convened and the swine flu program was officially begun with a presidential press conference.

"I have just concluded a meeting on a subject of vast importance to all Americans," the President began. "I have consulted with members of my Administration, with leading members of the health community, and with public health officials about the implications of this new appearance of swine flu. I have been advised that there is a very real possibility that unless we take effective counteractions, there could be an epidemic of this dangerous disease. At this time no one knows exactly how serious the threat could be. Nevertheless, we cannot afford to take a chance with the health of the Nation."[9]

The statement was carefully constructed. The President, for example, acknowledged that there would be mild reactions to the shot—"a very small price to pay for this vital protection." He hoped that Congress would act prior to its April recess. He noted that the best medical minds had been working on the problem and that the facts, although not suggesting alarm, did indicate "a need for immediate action."[10]

A week later, Congressman Rogers and Senator Kennedy convened their respective subcommittees to consider the President's request. Congressman Rogers explained the purpose of the hearings in his opening statement. The subject was of great concern because swine flu could very possibly appear "in such magnitude" as to represent a "clear and present threat to our citizens."[11] He discussed the history of swine flu and its severity and social costs. We are to consider spending $135 million: "I think it a wise investment in preventive medicine," he said.[12]

Senator Kennedy noted in his preamble that there was "nothing more frightening to a society than an epidemic."[13] The

President "has told us of the danger we face from this virus which is akin to the notorious swine flu of 1918-1919."[14]

As did Rogers, but far more explicitly, Kennedy intended to examine the "unparalleled opportunities" to improve the nation's health in other ways. There are children who have never been immunized, he said. Would it not be possible to immunize those children while they are standing in line waiting for their flu shots?[15]

Throughout the hearings, Senator Kennedy seemed preoccupied with the possibility of insuring that every child receive a full complement of shots for DPT, polio, and measles along with a swine flu inoculation. Children's immunizations were preventive medicine as much as were swine flu inoculations, he reasoned. Why not spend some more money and give our children a legacy to remember us by?[16]

Kennedy proved irrepressible in the hearings, asking about multiple injections and added monies to immunize children before he learned, as had Rogers a day earlier, that in addition to the logistical problems this posed, the safety and effectiveness of multiple inoculations had not yet been scientifically proven.[17]

Dr. Theodore Cooper, Assistant Secretary for Health, expressed the administration's concern. Before both subcommittees, he discussed the epidemiologic and immunological evidence which had led to the administration's "go" decision, the fact that they had consulted with national and international experts, and concluded that the only course of action was universal vaccination.[18]

Cooper and his colleagues chose their words carefully. The most Cooper would admit was that there was "a good likelihood" that the virus isolated at Fort Dix would result in an epidemic.[19] And Dr. Krause of the National Institute of Allergy and Infectious Diseases, testifying with Cooper, noted that the 1976 strain was "very similar" to the 1918 virus, but could not extrapolate to conclude that the 1976 strain was just as contagious or virulent.[20] The members of the subcommittees never asked the administration's scientists to discuss what was meant by "likelihood," "possibility," "probability," or any of the other technical nuances presented by the administration.

In his prepared remarks, which were submitted for the record but were not presented orally, Dr. Cooper also observed that the swine flu program "dwarfs in scope even the massive polio campaign which was undertaken in the 1950's after the licensure of Salk vaccine." The swine flu program, he said, would involve all segments of American society, as had the polio campaign, but to succeed would have to be planned, organized, and carried out in an extremely short period of time.[21]

During the course of the hearings in both House and Senate there was no further mention of polio; nor were there historical sojourns to consider other mass inoculation programs. The congressmen and senators of the subcommittees wanted to know about logistics. Can it be done? How quickly? How much would it cost? Certain medical questions were raised. Is the vaccine safe? How efficacious is it? Would there be side-effects? There was even a little humor. Dr. Harry Meyer, Director of the Bureau of Biologics of the FDA, commented on swine flu vaccine manufacture and noted that eggs were needed to grow the virus. Congressman Preyer of North Carolina, apologizing for his "poultry chauvinism," wanted to know if the eggs were fertilized. "I trust that our roosters are doing their bit for the country," he said.[22]

Mr. Joseph Stettler of the Pharmaceutical Manufacturers Association (PMA) told the subcommittees that firms were already experimenting with the production of the swine flu vaccine. He discussed timetables and informed the committee that it was impossible to predict whether or not 213 million doses of vaccine could be produced by early October. The PMA, however, could promise its most "diligent efforts."[23]

In addition to the scientific and production problems, Stettler admitted that there were also "major legal questions" to be answered, questions which "must be answered now," he said. The first issue was the need to provide a limited exemption for participating manufacturers from applicable antitrust laws. If a limited statutory exemption were not provided for participating companies, he said, they would be unable to discuss jointly such matters as optimum allocation of production quotas, matters relating to production and formulation techniques and joint research and testing.

The issue of liability was also raised by PMA. Since the manufacturers were to produce the vaccine in accordance with government specifications, and sell it to the government which would then dictate and coordinate its methods of distribution, it seemed "reasonable," said Stettler, for the government to indemnify the manufacturer for liabilities emanating from, or associated with, the use of the vaccine. Stettler pointed out that PMA was not suggesting that the manufacturer be indemnified against failure to produce "a quality vaccine," but that there were many problems associated with mass immunization programs, particularly in the light of a then recent legal decision which had held the manufacturer liable for an alleged injury in a community immunization program, even though the firm had had no connection with the program other than supplying the vaccine. The suit held that the company should have advised each person being immunized of the "potential harm" that the vaccine might cause.[24] Stettler argued that the manufacturer must have protection against such an "exaggerated interpretation of their responsibility in any mass inoculation program, especially one of the size and dimensions contemplated."

Again the questions from committee members concerned logistics, timetables, and costs, but eventually the legal issues were also considered. The questions concerning the legal aspects reveal an apparent lack of preparation on the part of the congressmen and senators in this phase of the history of the legislation. Congressman Waxman of California, for example, discussed PMA's justification for exemption from liability, but his questions were fuzzy and lacked authority.[25] He seemed satisfied with PMA's restatement of why they were seeking exemptions from liability and merely asked, without being able to extract any commitment, that PMA would be willing to consider a request to document the costs of the proposed federal program for a future Government Accounting Office report.[26]

Before the Senate subcommittee, Stettler again stated that the liability issue was so potentially enormous that PMA did not think that they "could obtain the necessary insurance coverage."[27] Senator Kennedy never asked for clarification or amplification of this startling statement.

The PMA, then, had clearly stated their needs, but at no time during the House or Senate subcommittee hearings was there any attempt to pursue any of these potential impediments to the national swine flu program. Only Dr. Cooper alluded to the potential problem, and hoped that the parties would get together and "make necessary sacrifices" to expedite the program "without any self-serving interests or profits to anyone."[28] In late March and early April, the administration certainly recognized the potential problems with respect to liability and insurance coverage, but, with the national interest at stake, simply did not believe that this potential for mischief would ever be fully realized.

If the Senate and House health subcommittees seemed to have "cast pseudo-light" on the issues, the hearings before the appropriations committees were even more perfunctory. On March 30, the House appropriations subcommittee unanimously approved the President's supplemental request, which now bore the title "House Joint Resolution 890," and, on April 2, the full committee reported the bill with the justification that "a potential health emergency exists which warrants immediate Federal aid and assistance."[29]

On April 5 the House of Representatives approved the resolution, and the Senate passed a similar measure on April 9, with some revisions. The House debate held few surprises, but before continuing it is neceesary to explain how this legislation differs from most other measures considered by the Congress.

The usual procedure is for a bill to be introduced, sent by the Parliamentarian to the appropriate committee or committees, hearings held, a bill reported from committee, debated on the floor of the Senate or House, and, if approved, subsequently considered by the appropriations committees, who in turn hold hearings and report their own bills, which are also debated on the floors of their respective chambers. The swine flu program, however, did not call for new authorizing legislation (for the administration contended that there already existed sufficient statutory authority), but rather for an emergency supplemental appropriation totalling $135 million to implement the program. The appropriations committees in both chambers quickly approved the resolution, but not before Congressman Rogers attempted to give the administration what it did not want: namely, authorizing legislation.

If the Congress approved of Rogers' strategy, which after all was the usual way of doing business in the Congress, then the Congress would be able to establish its priorities with regard to the proposed program rather than accept those of the administration. For example, in introducing his bill (H.R. 13012), which he brought to the House chamber under suspension of the rules the same day that the House was to debate the appropriations resolution, Rogers asked whether the administration had authority under existing statutes "to implement the program as they have contended?" He wondered "how much the vaccine would really cost?" And, picking up on testimony that he had taken from the Association of State and Territorial Health Officials, who had calculated that the program was severely underfinanced and that the state and local health departments would have to make up the difference by taking money from other necessary services, Rogers asked "how much the program would really cost the states?"

Rogers also wondered about liability insurance. Is there a need, he asked, "for immunization of the manufacturers against liability for reactions to the vaccine no matter how well made?"

There were other questions as well, none of which were answered; by and large, what Rogers really wanted was oversight control of the program and for the Secretary to make quarterly reports to the Congress on the administration of the program and the amount of funds expended.[30]

Rogers was denied his authorizing legislation because the Congress was persuaded that there was an urgency to the President's request. Even Congressman Michel of Illinois, who had always argued that the Congress "ought not be appropriating that for which [the Congress has] no authorizing legislation," accepted the position of the administration that swine flu was "a little different kind of situation . . . in view of the urgency of the matter and its unique character."[31] And so the House believed when it debated the bill later in the day. Only a few Congressmen opposed giving the administration what it wanted, and the measure passed, 354 to 12.[32]

Similarly, there was very little substantive debate in the Senate. Senator Magnuson introduced the measure with the qualification that "no one knows for sure whether the so-called swine flu will be a real threat." Nevertheless, it was a killer in 1918. If the scientific community, the President, and even our committee, are wrong, he said, then we might have wasted some scarce federal dollars that could have been used in other areas. "If the program is needed," however, "then the funds in the bill will save lives, prevent a great deal of human suffering, and save billions of dollars in medical costs."[33]

Senator Brooke also recommended passage of the supplemental appropriations bill. "I believe we cannot ignore [the scientific testimony we have heard]," he said. "We cannot take a chance with the health of our people. We must go forward with this program."[34] Senator Kennedy concurred. There may very well be some doubt that the epidemic will occur next Fall, he said, but "we cannot afford to take that chance with respect to protecting the health of the American people."[35]

Efforts by Senators Bumpers and Bayh on behalf of childhood immunizations[36] and by Senator Kennedy for increased appropriations for personnel and resources for FDA[37] were "for the record" only, but no one chose to champion the cause of the insurers or the manufacturers; nor was there any debate on the claim of the state and local health officers that their part of the appropriations package was inadequate.

The bill was an "emergency," said Magnuson;[38] it passed as introduced, 61 to 7.

On April 15 the President signed the emergency supplemental appropriations bill into law (P.L. 94–266) in the Oval Office. He referred to the legislation as "a timely response" to his request for "prompt congressional action."[39]

Unlike his statements of March 24 and 25, however, in which he carefully qualified his remarks about the virus, referring to it as *"very similar"* to one that caused the widespread and deadly flu epidemic of 1918–1919, he was much less guarded in his choice of words on April 15. There could be no turning back now as he declared that "this virus *was* the cause of a pandemic in 1918 and

1919 that resulted in over half a million deaths in the United States."[40]

The President, and the agency responsible for preparing the President's statement, were now committed and wedded to a course of action. The program was necessary because there would be a return of the 1918 virus—so testified the administration's scientists; so legislated the Congress; so proclaimed the President; so believed the American people. Or did they?

The truth of the matter is that no one really knew what the American people would believe. They had heard their President declare a virtual state of emergency, seen two of the most distinguished and venerable virologists in America at the President's side as he implored Americans to come forward to be inoculated, and heard nothing from the Congress. If America's scientists, the American Medical Association, American Academy of Family Practice, American Academy of Pediatrics, and the public health profession were all ready to cooperate with the President, as revealed in the hearings, why shouldn't the American people?

Events occurring in the spring and summer of 1976 were to make it virtually impossible for the people to know who or what to believe. And without that belief, the program never had a chance. In part, this is what happened. First, the New York *Times* declared that the entire affair was an election year gimmick. "A well-known advantage of being President before a Presidential election," observed the *Times,* "is the ability to use the office and its power to build a positive image before the voters." The *Times* questioned every one of the assumptions that were the basis for the program and disagreed with all of them, concluding that "The President's medical advisers seem to have panicked and to have talked him into a decision based on the worst assumptions about the still poorly known virus and the best assumptions about the vaccine."[41]

Rebuttal came from Dr. Edwin Kilbourne, one of this nation's most respected influenza virologists, who had advised the President in March. Kilbourne condemned the editorial for its "misstatements and ambiguities." Moreover, it was intemperate in "impugning the motives" of all parties involved. Kilbourne restated the assumptions upon which the program had been based and concluded that "not to proceed would represent an abrogation of responsibility to the public health."[42]

In June, the *Times* again editorialized. Despite months of surveillance there have been no additional human cases of swine flu, "let alone any signs of a deadly major epidemic which would justify the extraordinary program that President Ford—with the virtually unquestioning acquiescence of Congress—set in motion." Other industrial nations are "shrugging the whole thing off as another one of those incomprehensible American aberrations and overreactions that appear occasionally in political years," declared the *Times*.[43]

Kilbourne was again prompted to write. The *Times* has "assumed an awesome responsibility in its unmitigated hostility" to the swine flu program, Kilbourne began. Should swine flu appear in pandemic form next winter, Kilbourne asked, "will the *Times* be proud of its role in stimulating public doubt and discrediting the motives of those who (admitting the virus may not reappear) have advocated strong affirmative action to control a pandemic for the first time in history."[44]

On the same page, the *Times* rebutted Kilbourne in one of its nastier attacks. The program had been "sprung on the Nation," there had been "no public debate," the scientists had chosen the most "pessimistic possible projection from the scanty data," and moreover did so for their own "political advantage," and so on.[45]

The *Times* believed that its editorials should "stimulate public doubt." Having no power to command, they wrote, "our function is to stimulate thought and discussion."[46] Kilbourne must have thrown up his hands at that reasoning, for what he and his scientific colleagues in the administration and universities most feared appeared to be happening. The public was being asked to participate in a technical and scientific debate to which they had not been privy at the outset. Science was immutable and incorruptible, and here was the New York *Times* pointing out that scientists, examining the same data and evaluating the same evidence, disagreed with one another.[47] More damaging, perhaps, was the accusation that administration scientists were presenting the President with a course of action that would be uniquely to his political advantage. Scientists are supposed to eschew politics; the New York *Times* was implying that they were just like every other special interest group, except that they were more arrogant than most.

The second major problem to occur after the enactment of P.L. 94–266 concerned the insurance companies. For reasons that we have already discussed, the insurers dropped the other shoe in early summer and declared that they would no longer underwrite the coverage for the four firms producing the swine flu vaccine. One vaccine manufacturer had already curtailed production and the others appeared ready to follow.

To resolve the liability issue, in early June DHEW's legal staff prepared a draft proposal, which was introduced by Rogers on June 16. H.R. 14409 would have indemnified the manufacturers against claims attributable to inoculation with the swine flu vaccine, but would not apply to claims arising out of negligence on the part of the manufacturers.

Throughout the summer the House subcommittee found themselves in the unpleasant situation of not only having to decide whether or not a program was necessary on its scientific merits, but to report legislation which would break a legal impasse in as expeditious a manner as possible. No matter what the pressure from the administration, a program would not be possible without insurance, and insurance would not be possible without statutory authority provided by Congress.[48]

The problem was that all of the players refused to compromise. The vaccine producers, who ultimately agreed to produce a set limit of 90 million doses of the vaccine, wouldn't sell them to the government without liability insurance guarantees; the insurers wouldn't extend coverage without federal backing against losses; the subcommittee remained hostile to the idea of easing the government into the insurance business; and the administration refused to back down.[49]

On July 23, after yet another subcommittee donnybrook— this one before television cameras—Dr. Cooper, in the midst of his testimony, was handed a letter addressed to Congressman

Rogers, which he read into the record. It began, "Dear Paul," and was signed by the President.[50] Up to this moment the President had remained apart from the battle. At this late date, he had no other choice; things were getting out of hand.

Cooper read the letter aloud. It was cordial but shed no new light on the fundamental issues. The President reaffirmed his commitment to the program, reviewed the history of the decision (which by now was as familiar as a catechism), and asked for all parties "to work together to get on with the job." The threat of swine flu "is very genuine," he reiterated, and there is "no excuse to let this program bog down in petty wrangling."[51]

The President's letter poured oil over troubled waters, and for the rest of the session voices and tempers were lowered; but none of the fundamental issues were nearer solution.

If the New York *Times* and other media reactions raised doubts about the swine flu program, and the midsummer hearings revealed programmatic problems, then the final episode to be considered is the role played by accident. And this was the so-called Legionnaire's Disease, which mysteriously appeared in Philadelphia in late July.[52] It was a killer disease and, in effect, it "debogged" the program from its congressional mire.

The disease control specialists investigating the Philadelphia outbreak didn't know what to make of it. The media, however, was much more certain in their diagnosis, and the nation thought that swine flu was abroad in the land. So, too, did the House subcommittee. Thus, when it was learned that a new administration draft had been readied, which would protect the manufacturers from frivolous damage suits and which was acceptable to the manufacturers, insurers, and the department, Congressman Rogers grappled it to his bosom and rammed it through his subcommittee by a vote of 6 to 4.

Senator Kennedy introduced similar legislation in the Senate, but there were still snags. The first was that, by the end of the first week in August, the Philadelphia illness no longer appeared to be swine flu. Everyone breathed more easily, but congressional opponents to the measure had now time to regroup. A second snag was logistical. Congress was about to recess for the Republican national convention—again providing opponents with time for parliamentary maneuverings.

Time and politics, however, were on the side of the proponents of the measure. Urged by President Ford to protect the nation, and also urged to act by the Democratic leadership in the Congress so as not to give the Republicans before their convention a formidable weapon with which to denounce the Democratically controlled Congress,[53] Congress passed the liability package on August 10.

The Senate acted first. With Senator Kennedy at home nursing his chronic back problem,[54] Senator Javits and Senator Williams managed the bill on the floor of the Senate. The previous night the staffs of the House and Senate subcommittees, together with representatives of the administration, prepared a substitute measure to the administration's draft bill (H.R. 15050). This new Senate bill (S. 3735) was first sent to the Appropriations Committee where Senator McClellan, by agreement with Senator Kennedy, reported the bill "without prejudice or any specific recommendation."[55] Javits then moved that the bill be brought up for debate and, without objection, the bill was on its own, now in the hands of one of the Senate's most gifted debaters.

Javits began with a review of the liability issue and itemized the sections of the new authorizing legislation. The fundamental thrust of the bill had not changed—the government would assume liability for personal injuries connected with the program, would be subject to claims and suits under the Federal Tort Claims Act, and would have a right to sue the program participant where the United States had paid a claim based on the manufacturer's or provider's negligence—but the compromise measure also included important sections on informed consent, the return of monies to the United States on excess manufacturer's profits if contracts were renegotiated, and studies which the Secretary would be required to conduct. The bill was not to become precedent; it was rather an expedient, a one-year stop-gap measure to meet a national emergency.[56]

Javits also alluded to the Philadelphia episode, not as he said to invoke the specter of swine flu, but rather to have the Senate consider the "suddenness with which a terrible disease can strike." How guilty the Congress would be, he said, "if having been forewarned by our scientists, we had not heeded their advice and had been caught flatfooted and completely unprepared." That is "the lesson" of Philadelphia, he concluded.[57]

Senator Taft then hoped that the liability section would not become a precedent;[58] Senator Williams urged the passage of the measure because in a sense it was "pioneering" new territory;[59] and Senator Allen introduced an amendment (subsequently withdrawn) which would have assured that the program was totally voluntary (which it already was).[60]

While the Senate bill was being debated and approved, Paul Rogers and his staff aides set up a command field post in the House cloakroom. They kept in touch with Senate staffers by telephone to see if any changes would have to be made in the now identical bills. The House bill, which had been approved by Rogers' subcommittee, had never been approved by its parent, the Interstate and Foreign Commerce Committee. Earlier in the day, Harley Staggers, chairman of the full committee, had waited in vain for a quorum. Opponents to the measure had decided that the best way to derail the program would be to keep the bill from coming to the floor. Rogers, however, had a fall-back strategy. As soon as the Senate had passed its version of the bill, he brought it to the House Rules Committee, pleaded the "national interest," and was able to win the approval of the Rules Committee to bring the measure up for debate. But not before the rule itself was debated.

And it was quite a debate.

Richmond Flowers of Georgia thought the proposal a rush job. What will happen if the bill passes, he said, is to "let our Government, your Government and mine and therefore the people we represent, to become the target of lawsuits in every U.S. district court in the land."[61] Congressman Moss of California pointed out that the House was being "stampeded" into considering a bill based on a "national emergency" which no longer existed.[62] Congressman Dingell of Michigan thought that the manner in which the measure had been brought to the floor was "irresponsible." The bill was not insurance, nor was it a guarantee. "It is an absolute unbridled, total unlimited assumption of responsibility and liability," he said.[63]

Rogers rebutted the arguments. He invoked the name of science ("The experts, the scientists, have told us . . ."), raised the specter of pandemics ("Do the Members know what happened in 1918 and 1968?"), and brought forth a hitherto unknown document from the chairman of the Judiciary Committee, Peter Rodino, which Rogers contended supported the measure. "I hold no brief for the insurance companies," Rogers concluded.[64] They have not "met their responsibilities," but as the Congress does not license them, "we cannot make them go out and insure somebody if they do not want to."[65]

The question to debate the rule was called and the motion carried, 272 to 76. Rogers then called from the Speaker's desk the Senate-passed substitute (S. 3735), and the debate began afresh.

Rogers especially debated Waxman, who was now the most vigorous opponent of the program. Waxman argued that the bill would relieve the drug manufacturers and the insurance industry from their responsibility of being legally and financially liable for their product. The insurance industry, he contended, was seeking to be relieved from responsibility in areas of coverage where they do not make "big profits." Although this may not be the case with this program, he said, it will have the effect of setting a precedent for future programs. Today it is swine flu, tomorrow it may be polio and measles vaccine and even malpractice insurance. "We are being used, Mr. Speaker," he said. "I think we are making a big mistake."[66]

Congressman Hungate of Missouri was similarly opposed because the full Judiciary Committee had not reviewed the bill. Mr. Rodino's views were "not always totally encompassing without the benefit of the views of the whole committee," he said.[67] Congressman Carter, the only physician on the health subcommittee, joined in the debate, contemplated the potential swine flu "holocaust," and rattled off statistics about the number of deaths that had been caused by the 1918 swine flu epidemic in his home state of Kentucky.[68]

Congressman Frenzel of Minnesota then summarized the debate. He said that "the bill made him nervous." Certainly, "we are making a mistake," he said.

> But we really have no choice. The drug companies won't produce vaccine without some relief of their legal liability. I can't blame them for their unwillingness to accept unlimited liability. Therefore, we have to pass this bill if we want an anti-swine flu program. If we had more time, we might be able to devise another system under which we can administer the vaccine. We do not have time. We must support this bill.[69]

The question was then called and the measure passed, 250 to 83.

Those who opposed the measure were a misalliance of conservatives, liberals, and just about all the members of the Black Caucus. The Black Caucus took no concerted stand on the issue, however. They did not oppose it because it did nothing to immunize the children of the inner city. Rather they opposed it for the same reasons as did liberals and conservatives; namely, that the insurance companies were getting a free ride.

In the presence of Secretary Matthews, Congressman Carter, Dr. Cooper, and an audience composed of physicians and media representatives, the President signed the "National Swine Flu Immunization Program of 1976" (S. 3735) into law (P.L. 94–380) on August 12. The President described the program and its mechanisms to protect the manufacturers. He said that the vaccine, "which will afford millions of Americans protection against an outbreak of swine flu in the winter," would now be made available as quickly as possible. And he concluded: "I say again, I am grateful that the Congress did take this action so this program could continue."[70]

The President's sense of relief, however, was very short-lived. What happened between September and December 1976—the scientific debate about dose rates and antibody levels, the implementation problems at the state and local levels, the predictable but untimely deaths in Pittsburgh, the unexpected deaths owing to Guillain-Barré, and the eventual suspension of the program in December—must be told at another time.[71] But here are some impressions and interpretations that we might wish to consider.

First, I see no personal goodness or badness in the events I have related. What I do see is men and institutions trapped in a predicament with right and wrong on both sides and the U.S. Congress caught in the middle.[72]

Congress grappled with issues that it is simply not equipped to understand. Deciding to gamble that the swine flu threat was genuine, it had little to debate other than issues that lawyers do understand—torts, liability, profits, and "flim-flam." Yet even here the Congress provided no leadership. For over two months during the summer, the Congress remained apart from the liability issue which had actually emerged as early as March 31. It was the administration's problem, Congress seemed to say; let them resolve the difficulties. Of course, it was everybody's problem. For over ten years, there has been a steady attrition of specific pharmaceutical manufacturers from the entire field of biologics. A relatively low profit margin, high production risks, increasing costs of research and development, difficulties in clinical testing, and stringent governmental standards have all been cited as formidible constraints to private investment.[73] Since the Kefauver-Harris amendments, the drug companies have believed that they have been the Congress' whipping boy.[74] Now they were saying that they had had enough. Liability *was* an issue. Resolve it by revising the tort laws, by reinsurance, by a modification of the Price-Anderson Act (under which the government indemnifies licencees and contractors working on federal and private nuclear projects),[75] or with mechanisms set forth in P.L. 94–380. But do something; or produce your own biologics.

The problem was lack of time to do anything constructive. The most troubling aspects about Congress are the short attention span of its members and its full legislative agenda. Congress provides a forum for the issues, invites competing interests to present viewpoints at its hearings, but misses too many opportunities to take issues to bits. No sooner is swine flu passed than tax reform emerges, which gives way to clean air, which gives way to medical manpower, and so on. One cluster of Congressmen and their staff massage one issue, and with equal vigor, enthusiasm, and superficiality slip off to massage another of equal magnitude.

The second problem was that the scientists who advised the President were similarly captured by events and data which could have led only to what Kilbourne himself called a "$135 million gamble"[76] and CDC a "calculated gamble."[77] Decisions of this type, wrote Franz Ingelfinger, "unavoidably are made under circumstances in which the principles of Pascal's Wager predominate."[78] None of the scientists were able to assure the President that a viral flu epidemic would not rage in 1976–1977, and few of the experts were able to suggest an alternative and reasonably effective prophylactic measure. If the vaccine were given and nothing happened, no one would be blamed and the scientists and the President would be praised.[79] But, if the vaccination program had not been recommended and an epidemic occurred, who then would want to be anywhere near where that decision had been made? Sabin said it more succinctly, "We were damned if we did and damned if we didn't."[80] CDC said it more prosaically, "Better to have an immunization program without an epidemic, than an epidemic without an immunization program."[81]

The Congress took testimony from Sabin, Salk, and the administration's scientists.[82] They learned facts about the virus and vaccine and had what amounted to a cram course in influenza immunology. In late June and July, they learned from Salk that the program should proceed as had been planned, no matter what had been published in the New York *Times* or the *Lancet;*[83] they learned from Sabin that the program should be modified, only high risks vaccinated and the remainder of the vaccine stockpiled; and they learned from the administration's scientists why stockpiling the vaccine was a bankrupt policy no matter what the World Health Organization had recommended in April.[84] There were no other appeals to higher scientific authority, because there was no one else to appeal to! Turning inward, then, Congress avoided the scientific issues it neither comprehended nor wished to comprehend and made a political decision.

Third, the role of the media must be considered. The *Times,* for example, "stimulated thought and discussion" on the issue, but they also "stimulated public doubt."[85] In January of this year, in yet another philippic, the New York *Times,* for example, observed that "Public health is inevitably bound to public faith and that our government was ill enough without this medical venture."[86] The *Times* scratched the surface of our health bureaucracy and found an administration and Congress, as they wrote, lacking in "the scientific sophistication to be able to put biological reality before political expediency."[87] It was as if, in this ill-fated program, they had found a single public health equivalent to the Bay of Pigs, Gulf of Tonkin, and Watergate.

A group of distinguished scientists, including the Nobel laureate John Enders, recently rebutted the *Times,* calling their comments and editorials "one-sided interpretations of the actual events,"[88] but the paper never relented from its position that the policy decision had been formed hastily, and that the government "scorned the few voices that expressed skepticism and sought to raise questions about the program."[89]

The administration replied to this accusation at an oversight hearing in December, when the program had been suspended owing to Guillain-Barré. When asked by Senator Kennedy what they would have done differently if they had it to do over again, Dr. Cooper replied that "the most important thing" would have been a "more comprehensive widespread discussion with all sectors of the public . . . so that everybody could understand what the scientific information was and what the anticipated types of problems were."[90] The National Immunization Conference held in November 1976 was an example of how the government sought to widen the debate, but it was nine months too late.

The short and not so very happy life history of the national swine influenza program has already become a classic health policy case study because the elements of policy and politics are so illustratively intertwined. However, to derive conclusions from the events is not so simple. If one wishes to find heroes and villains in the piece, they will certainly be found; if one wishes to view the Congress as a moribund or trifling institution, there is abundant evidence to do so; if one wishes to interpret the action of the administration and its scientists as being politically motivated and self-serving, he will find circumstantial evidence to support the theory; and if one wishes to view the President's decision as being based upon some real or imagined bicentennial or electoral bonanza, he will also find evidence to support that thesis. But he will also find, as others have found, men and institutions "muddling through,"[91] making their decisions hastily and "under conditions of chronic obscurity," where chance, accident, confusion, and stupidity play a larger role than certitude or calculation.[92]

If anything positive emerges from the events of 1976, it will be the creation of a National Immunization Commission,[93] charged with making long-range plans and serving as the arbiter of last resort; the appropriation of more money to immunize children;[94] the statutory resolution of the concerns expressed by the manufacturers and the insurers; the development of a national immunization program; the hiring of congressional staff with prerequisite medical and scientific sophistication;[95] and a pervasive understanding by all concerned parties that the public must in some way participate in the decisions of its government.[96]

If the events of 1976 are not to recur, then the Congress and the administration had better ensure that these issues are addressed now.

References

1. See, for example, U.S. Congress, Senate, Committee on Labor and Public Welfare, *Legislative Review Activity*, 95th Cong., 1st sess., 1977, S. Rept. 95–80, March 31, 1977, pp. 29–43.

2. Walter R. Dowdle, "The swine flu vaccine program," *American Society for Microbiology News*, May 1977, *43:* 5, p. 243.

3. A copy of this memorandum has been deposited in the "Contemporary Medical Care and Health Policy Collection," Manuscripts and Archives, Yale University Library, New Haven, Connecticut.

4. *Ibid.*, p. 2.

5. *Ibid.*, p. 4.

6. *Ibid.*, pp. 4–5.

7. *Ibid.*, pp. 5–7.

8. *Ibid.*, p. 8.

9. *Weekly Compilation of Presidential Documents,* March 29, 1976, *12:* 3, pp. 483–484.

10. *Ibid.,* p. 484.

11. U.S. Congress, House, Committee on Interstate and Foreign Commerce, Subcommittee on Health and the Environment, *Hearings on Proposed National Swine Flu Vaccination Program,* 94th Cong., 2nd sess., March 31, 1976, p. 1.

12. *Ibid.,* pp. 1–2.

13. U.S. Congress, Senate, Committee on Labor and Public Welfare, Subcommittee on Health, *Hearings on Swine Flu Immunization Program,* 94th Cong., 2nd sess., April 1, 1976, p. 1.

14. *Ibid.*

15. *Ibid.*

16. *Ibid.,* pp. 2, 9, 13, 68.

17. *Ibid.,* pp. 9–10. See also House hearings (March 31, 1976) *op. cit.,* pp. 17–19, 46, 57–58.

18. House hearings (March 31, 1976), *op. cit.,* pp. 7–33; Senate hearings (April 1, 1976), *op. cit.,* pp. 6–53.

19. House hearings (March 31, 1976), *op. cit.,* p. 8.

20. *Ibid.,* p. 13.

21. *Ibid.,* p. 10.

22. *Ibid.,* pp. 14–15. Chairman Rogers then revealed that he had "just been handed a note that, even though we may give much credit to the rooster, don't forget the hens in this date and age." p. 15.

23. *Ibid.,* p. 34.

24. *Ibid.,* pp. 33–36, 40–42; Senate hearings (April 1, 1976), *op. cit.,* pp. 71–83.

25. House hearings (March 31, 1976), *op. cit.,* pp. 40–42.

26. *Ibid.,* pp. 41–42.

27. Senate hearings (April 1, 1976), *op. cit.,* p. 73.

28. House hearings (March 31, 1976), *op. cit.,* p. 8.

29. U.S. Congress, House, Committee on Appropriations, *Emergency Supplemental Appropriations, 1976,* 94th Cong., 2nd sess., H. Rept. 94-1004, April 2, 1976, p. 3.

30. U.S. Congress, House, *Congressional Record*, April 5, 1976, pp. 2861–2865.

31. *Ibid.*, p. 2863.

32. *Ibid.*, pp. 2871–2875.

33. U.S. Congress, Senate, *Congressional Record*, April 9, 1976, pp. 5347–5348.

34. *Ibid.*, p. 5353.

35. *Ibid.*, p. 5355.

36. *Ibid.*, pp. 5348, 5350–5351.

37. *Ibid.*, pp. 5355–5356.

38. *Ibid.*, p. 5349.

39. *Weekly Compilation of Presidential Documents*, April 19, 1976, *12*: 16, p. 656.

40. *Ibid.* [My italics.]

41. N.Y. *Times*, April 6, 1976.

42. *Ibid.*, April 14, 1976.

43. *Ibid.*, June 8, 1976.

44. *Ibid.*, August 9, 1976.

45. *Ibid.*

46. *Ibid.*

47. *Ibid.* For further information about scientific validity and scientific advice, see S.J. Reiser, "Smoking and health; the Congress and causality," in S. Lakoff (ed.), *Knowledge and Power: Essays on Science and Government* (N.Y.: Free Press, 1966), pp. 293–311; M.J. Mahoney, *The Scientist: Anatomy of the Truth Merchant* (Cambridge: Ballinger, 1976); and I.T. Mitroff, *The Subjective Side of Science* (N.Y.: Elsevier, 1974).

48. U.S. Congress, *Congressional Record*, August 26, 1976, p. E4699.

49. *Washington Report on Medicine and Health*, July 26, 1976, *30*: 30, p. 1.

50. U.S. Congress, House, Committee on Interstate and Foreign Commerce, Subcommittee on Health and the Environment, *Supplemental Hearings on Swine Flu Immunization Program*, 94th Cong., 2nd sess., June 28, July 20, 23, and September 13, 1976, pp. 265–267.

51. *Ibid.*, p. 267.

52. See Barbara J. Culliton's "Legion fever: postmortem of an investigation that failed," *Science*, December 2, 1976, *194:* 4269, pp. 1025–1027 and "Legion fever: 'failed' investigation may be successful after all," *ibid.*, February 4, 1977, *195:* 4277, pp. 469–470.

53. *Washington Report on Medicine and Health*, August 16, 1976, *30:* 33, p. 1.

54. As is often the case, members often submit material for the record which appears in the *Congressional Record* even though they were not present during the debate. If one chose to read the *Record*, they would have learned that Kennedy excoriated the insurers. Their position was one of "intransigence." They had held the program "hostage." They had acted "precipitously and abruptly" and were threatening to act in a similar manner with respect to polio and measles immunizations. They had shown "both a cupidity and inexcusable lack of social obligation to the needs of the American people." And, to show how really mad he was, he promised to introduce an amendment to repeal the special insurance exemptions from the McCarran-Ferguson antitrust act! See *Record*, August 10, 1976, pp. 14116–14117.

55. U.S. Congress, Senate, Committee on Appropriations, *National Swine Flu Immunization Program of 1976*, 94th Cong., 2nd sess., S. Rept. 94–1147, August 10, 1976, p. 1.

56. U.S. Congress, Senate, *Congressional Record*, August 10, 1976, pp. 14108–14109.

57. *Ibid.*, p. 14109.

58. *Ibid.*, p. 14110.

59. *Ibid.*, p. 14113.

60. *Ibid.*, pp. 14117–14118.

61. U.S. Congress, House, *Congressional Record*, August 10, 1976, p. 8644.

62. *Ibid.*

63. *Ibid.*

64. *Ibid.*, p. 8645.

65. *Ibid.*

66. *Ibid.*, pp. 8649–8650.

67. *Ibid.*, p. 8651.

68. *Ibid.,* p. 8652.

69. *Ibid.,* p. 8654.

70. *Weekly Compilation of Presidential Documents,* August 16, 1976, *12:* 33, pp. 1256–1257.

71. See Dowdle, *op. cit.;* Jonas Salk, "The ultimate flu vaccine," *Saturday Review,* November 27, 1976, pp. 18–19; Richard Restak, "The great vaccination flap," *ibid.,* pp. 6–11; George A. Silver, "Lessons of the swine flu debacle," *The Nation,* February 12, 1977, pp. 166–169; "Swine flu: did Uncle Sam buy a pig in a poke?" *Consumer Reports,* September 1976, pp. 495–498; Lawrence Wright, "Sweating out the swine flu scare," *New Times,* May 11, 1976, pp. 28–38; Thomas O'Toole, "Why the swine flu program failed," Washington *Post,* January 30, 1977, p. C3; Stephen C. Schoenbaum, et al, "The swine-influenza decision," *New England Journal of Medicine,* September 30, 1976, *295:* 14, pp. 759–765; Louis Weinstein, "Influenza—1918, a revisit?," *ibid.,* May 6, 1976, *294:* 19, pp. 1058–1060; Alfred M. Prince, "Our last vaccine?," *Science,* March 25, 1977, *195:* 4284, p. 1287; Edwin D. Kilbourne, "National immunization for pandemic influenza," *Hospital Practice,* June 1976, pp. 15–21; and five superb articles by Philip M. Boffey, "Anatomy of a decision: how the nation declared war on swine flu," *Science,* May 14, 1976, *192:* 4240, pp. 636–641; "Swine flu vaccination campaign: the scientific controversy mounts," *ibid.,* August 13, 1976, *193,* pp. 559–563; "Swine flu vaccine: a component is missing," *ibid.,* September 24, 1976, *193,* pp. 1224–1225; "Guillain-Barré: rare disease paralyzes swine flu campaign," *ibid.,* January 14, 1977, *195,* pp. 155–159; and "Soft evidence and hard sell," *N.Y. Times Magazine,* September 5, 1976, pp. 8 ff. Other articles, monographs, and anthologies will doubtless follow these, lending credence to Tom Wicker's epigrammatic conclusion about personalities and circumstances in politics, that ". . . if someone else would tell these stories differently, that is only to be welcomed. Who would wish for a single, authorized version of the endless adventure?" See Tom Wicker, *JFK and LBJ: The Influence of Personality Upon Politics* (Baltimore: Penguin Books, 1968), p. 21.

72. This is a paraphrase of a sentence appearing in Arthur Schlesinger Jr.'s essay, "The historian as participant," *Daedulus,* Spring 1971, *100:* 2, pp. 345–346.

73. JRB Associates, Inc., "National Immunization Work Group on Production and Supply," *Reports and Recommendations of the Na-*

tional Immunization [Conference] Work Groups, March 15, 1977, Submitted to the Office of the Assistant Secretary for Health (Virginia: JRB Associates, Inc., 1977), p. 1.

74. See, for example, Estes Kefauver, *In a Few Hands; Monopoly Power in America* (Baltimore: Penguin Books, 1965), pp. 8–79, and Milton Silverman and Philip R. Lee, *Pills, Profits and Politics* (Berkeley: Univ. of Calif. Press, 1974).

75. House hearings (March 31, 1976), p. 41. For additional information about Price-Anderson, see U.S. Congress, Joint Committee on Atomic Energy, *Hearings, Governmental Indemnity and Reactor Safety*, 85th Cong., 1st sess., May 25, 26, 27, 1957, and either H. Rept. No. 435 or S. Rept. No. 296, *Amending the Atomic Energy Act of 1954 . . .*, Joint Committee, May 9, 1957.

76. Edwin D. Kilbourne, "A $135-million gamble," *Natural History*, June-July 1976, *75:* 6, pp. 39–41.

77. Connecticut State Department of Health, *Influenza in the United States; Rationale for Mass Immunizations in 1976* (Hartford: State Department of Public Health, 1976), p. 11. CDC provided all state health departments with the narrative for this and similar publications provided by the National Influenza Immunization Program.

78. Franz Ingelfinger, "Thou shalt be vaccinated," *New England Journal of Medicine*, May 6, 1976, *294:* 19, p. 1060.

79. *Ibid.*

80. House hearings (June 28, 1976), *op. cit.,* p. 62.

81. *Influenza in the United States, op. cit.,* p. 11.

82. House (June 28, July 20, 23) and Senate (August 5, 1976) hearings, *op. cit.*

83. The *Lancet* published three pieces on swine flu in July. The papers disputed the seriousness of the threat and the efficacy of the vaccines. Six volunteers, for example, were inoculated with the new virus; all became infected but their reactions were mild. More important, however, was the observation that the virus neither spread when introduced into a closed community of young people nor replaced A-Victoria as the prevalent strain. See A.S. Beare and J.W. Craig, "Virulence for man of a human influenza-A virus antigenically similar to 'classical' swine viruses," pp. 4–5; "Planning for pandemics," pp. 25–26; and Charles Stuart-Harris, "Swine influenza virus in man; zoonosis or human

pandemic?," pp. 31–32, all in *The Lancet,* July 3, 1976, *2:* 7975. None
of these papers were appended to House or Senate subcommittee
hearings.

84. See World Health Organization, *Weekly Epidemiological Record,*
"Influenza," April 15, 1976, No. 16, pp. 123–134. See, also, A.B. Sabin's, "Washington and the Flu," N.Y. *Times,* November 5, 1976, and
"Swine flu: what happened," *The Sciences,* March/April 1977, *17:* 2,
pp. 14 ff.

85. N.Y. *Times,* August 9, 1976.

86. *Ibid.,* January 3, 1977.

87. Harry Schwartz, "The swine flu fiasco," N.Y. *Times,* December 21,
1976.

88. "Swine flu: in defense of the Administration's decision to vaccinate,"
ibid, January 10, 1977. Other than Enders, the letter was signed by T.C.
Chalmers, M.D. (Mount Sinai School of Medicine), R.H. Ebert, M.D.
(Harvard), J.T. Grayson, M.D. (University of Washington), Abraham
Lilienfield, M.D. (Johns Hopkins), and D.D. Rutstein, M.D. (Har-
vard).

89. Schwartz, *op. cit.*

90. U.S. Congress, Senate, Committee on Labor and Public Welfare,
Subcommittee on Health, *Hearings on Suspension of the Swine Flu
Immunization Program, 1976.* 94th Cong., 2nd sess., December 17,
1976, p. 11.

91. See Charles E. Lindblom, "The science of 'muddling through',"
Public Administration Review, Spring 1959, *19:* 2, pp. 79–88.

92. Schlesinger, *op. cit.,* p. 354. Schlesinger's full quote is: "General
George Marshall used to say that battlefield decisions were taken under
conditions of 'chronic obscurity'—that is, under excessive pressure on
the basis of incomplete and defective information. This is probably the
character of most critical decisions in the field of public policy. The
eyewitness historian tends to preserve the felt texture of events and to
recognize the role of such elements as confusion, ignorance, chance,
and sheer stupidity."

93. JRB Associates, Inc., *op. cit.*

94. N.Y. *Times,* April 7, 11, and 12, 1977. See, also, Joseph A. Califano,
Jr., "Address to Second National Immunization Conference," *HEW
News,* April 6, 1977.

95. In 1976, the Senate staff responsible for the swine flu legislation were
    non-physicians; the House staff did include one physician, with four
    years of congressional experience and one year of postgraduate medical
    training.

96. "National Immunization Work Group on Health Information and
    Public Awareness," JRB Associates, Inc., *op cit.*, pp. 1–12.

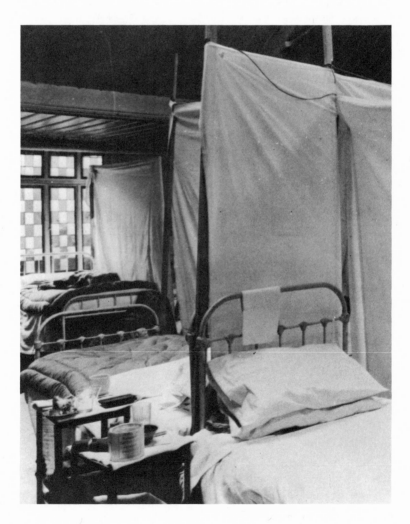

Epilogue—
The Costs and Benefits of the
National Immunization Program
of 1976

JUNE E. OSBORN

When the full gaze of the Fourth Estate is caught and focused, the effect is somewhat like the searchlight scan of a prison yard: Any creature that so much as moves or casts a shadow within its glare becomes the object of such gaudy attention that innocent and guilty alike become befuddled. From the day that Gerald Ford entered the influenza drama bringing in his wake all the candle-power that automatically follows the American Presidency, the opportunity was essentially lost for public health leaders to achieve a careful, rational education of the consuming public about the "swine flu" immunization decision and program.

Careful, scrupulous professional science writers for the nation's leading newspapers and periodicals had already spent long hours in briefing and study to learn the complex background of influenza virology and epidemiology that would enable them to convey an accurate risk/benefit analysis to their readers. Indeed, many excellent articles had been written prior to and in fact after the President's announcement of the swine flu campaign. Actually the story in the summer of 1976 was extremely undramatic, for almost nothing *had* happened; only what *might* happen made potentially interesting reading.

The simple facts were rather dull. We were coming to the end of a "pandemic era," and it was about time for a new influenza A variant to surface and infect a fresh world of susceptibles. A new influenza strain *had* emerged late in the 1975–1976 flu season, and its late appearance might not only explain why it caused just one identifiable outbreak but might also give the precious lead time which had been unavailable or lost in previous pandemic year vaccine production efforts. Even duller were the legally mandated routines which had to be conducted before a new vaccine could be produced in any quantity; although the production method of the "swine flu" vaccine was identical to that used in all recent influenza vaccine production programs, the virus was technically new and, therefore, the final product had to undergo careful testing to establish dose, efficacy, safety, and so on. This procedure is standard and is in fact part of why it takes several months to prepare for mass production of influenza vaccines. The methodical testing of serums before and after test immunization and the analysis of antibody response in different categories of age, sex, and other characteristics of the volunteer vaccinees was already under way under the supervision of Dr. Harry M. Meyer, Jr. and the staff of the FDA's Bureau of Biologics; the results were as exciting as a computer printout. The vaccine worked well, and a dose could be identified for individuals over the age of 25 which yielded 90 percent seroconversions (i.e., satisfactory antibody responses) while only 2 percent or less of the recipients had any side effects such as sore arms or brief fevers.

Somewhat surprisingly, the age group under 25 presented a slight problem, for a dose sufficient to reliably elicit an antibody response also caused febrile responses with a frequency deemed unacceptable. However, an alternative was available in the form of a so-called "split product" vaccine—in the preparation of which the killed, purified influenza virus particles were partially disassembled chemically. This preparation was significantly less toxic and, when given in two divided doses a month apart, was equally satisfactory as a vaccine for the under-25 age group. The press tried to make something of the multiple dosage schedules, but this issue was certainly not the stuff of which good copy is made, for it should surprise no one that a dose of *anything*— vaccine, antibiotic, or aspirin—might have to be modulated according to the age of the recipient; and despite the perfection demanded by 1976 consumers, very few products in that year were

as much as 90 percent likely to do what was claimed for them.
Even the best of the miraculous vaccines of the two preceding
decades were only about 95 percent effective, leaving a small
residue of vaccinees whose failure to respond presumably reflected the pure realities of biologic variation.

And so the science of the new influenza vaccine moved
systematically and smoothly forward without any new—much
less interesting—surprises. The bare facts could have been briefly
and easily reported, and since no one was to be *required* to
participate in the program (which was often overlooked in the
hue and cry) consumers could draw their own risk/benefit analysis and gamble either for antibody protection or for a quiet
influenza season, as they saw fit.

However, another kind of science—epidemiology—was going to need presentation to the public. Biologic variation is truly
at the heart of large-scale public health events, and a mass campaign that would touch an entire population in a brief interval
raised some difficult issues that were acutely evident to epidemiologists at the very moment of the program's inception.

The central problem was as follows: It had become custom-
ary to attempt as broad an assessment as possible of the adverse
effects of *any* vaccine by tentatively scoring against the vaccine
any illness that occurred in the month that followed its inoculation administration. Clearly this was an overly conservative measure of vaccine side effects but, since it erred on the side of safety, it
was a well-established surveillance practice. Now, if you record
all the illnesses and other unpleasant events that befall a substantial fraction of 200,000,000 people in any four-week interval, you
will have a catalogue of every possible permutation of human
illness and misery—not all of which can by any means be causally
explained. Regarded in that way, it became obvious to epidemiologist and intelligent layman alike that restrained assessment and
reporting of purported flu vaccine side effects would be essential
to avoid the potential panic of a false association. The true
challenge to the Fourth Estate lay, therefore, less in teaching the
science of influenza virology and immunology than in establishing an appreciation of numerators and denominators, of risks and

benefits, of indeterminate causality, and—most fundamental—of the right of highly trained scientists to be *uncertain* without losing their credibility as experts.

But such restraint did not appeal to the hordes of journalists who were *not* scientific or medical writers; for much better—and much more—copy could be written about the "human interest story" and the possibility of exposé. In a country where the stifling of dissent is abhorrent, dissenters can always be found. The initial "go" decision to proceed with the mass immunization program had already essentially been made by dozens of the government's scientific and medical advisers by the time it was taken to the arena of the Oval Office. The experts had nothing to gain by their recommendation (and, as they learned, plenty to lose—at least in the currency of peace and quiet during the months that followed) and had spent days of public debate in workshops sifting and weighing the dry facts to achieve a balanced plan. Of those that received the full briefing, none dissented loudly—and most were the sort of people who would not have been shy had they had serious reservations or concern.

But a few dissident scientists who felt excluded from the chosen circle of advisers set up a chorus of howls: A rip-off was in progress! A new, unknown, untested, probably unsafe, surely ineffectual vaccine against a non-existent virus was being foisted on an unsuspecting public! Worse yet, they pointed out (in a master stroke of clang association certain to create public confusion) that the virus being used to prepare the vaccine was a *recombinant*! The A/New Jersey/76 isolate had, in fact, been "recombined" in the laboratory with an older influenza A strain to improve its efficiency at growing in eggs rather than in humans—a practice that had been used in the past to increase the speed with which vaccine could finally be mass-produced. The cleverly accusing use of the word "recombinant," however, invoked all the specters of an extremely current, hot, and scientifically totally unrelated argument concerning "recombinant DNA" research.

Lest I seem unfair in reporting the dissent against the swine flu program, I hasten to comment that dissent grew in responsible quarters as well. In particular it was argued that perhaps the vaccine should only be produced and stockpiled until the next sign of potential pandemic was evident; that argument grew easier and louder as months passed without the reappearance of the "swine flu." But the unrestrained clamor from a remarkably small group of all-out critics was like the moving shadow in the prison yard: All searchlights pivoted and focused.

And so it was that, when the epidemic season was under way, the expert advisers were chastened for having been "wrong"! There was no pandemic as promised! Yet no one had promised a pandemic or even asserted the strong likelihood of one. Simply, the elements were at hand, and the possibility of a major, preventable influenza outbreak was *finite*.

When three elderly and ill vaccine recipients in Pittsburgh died within hours of receiving their flu shots, vigorous governmental investigation was appropriately launched and conducted to be sure the vaccine was not causally implicated; nevertheless, common sense was—or should have been—quickly reassuring, for hundreds of others received shots in the same clinic on the same day without misadventure, and the three who died had received the vaccine early in the program by virtue of their advanced age and infirmity. Again the cries of "I told you so" came loudly from the dissenters.

The swine flu program was finally slain and buried by an obscure entity called the Guillain-Barré syndrome. That form of ascending paralysis, like all other neurologic diseases, was a terrifying experience for those who experienced it, although it was usually temporary in its paralytic effects. Indeed, it had much the same physical and psychological effect as had poliomyelitis in the old days—but the public had forgotten polio. Like many other neurologic syndromes, its cause was unknown and had been much researched. It is relatively rare and had not been on the list of diseases physicians were required to report to CDC, so that its exact incidence was unknown. Given its rarity, however, many biomedical scientists assumed that, if an infectious agent were involved, it had to be only part of the cause: Anything that was a mass experience and/or contagious ought to occur much more commonly. In the past, epidemiologists and neurologists had tried to identify distinctive antecedent events which might lend a clue to environmental factors contributing to this unusual paralytic syndrome.

When cases of Guillain-Barré's ascending paralysis began to appear in the late fall of 1976, the surveillance system for untoward results of the flu program was active at an unprecedented level of sensitivity, and the response was brisk. CDC investigated, found a statistical association between flu immunization and subsequent occurrence of the syndrome, and Assistant Secretary for Health Theodore Cooper abruptly halted the immunization program. The decision was not difficult, for by then the flu season was well under way and was very quiet indeed; only sporadic cases of flu-like disease were occurring and many of those appeared to be caused by influenza B, which was not included in the vaccine formulation for the mass campaign. It took weeks of sleuthing and analysis to find out what the Guillain-Barré association was: Whereas the ordinary citizen had had one chance in a million of contracting Guillain-Barré syndrome in the winter of 1976-1977, those who received their "swine flu shot" had that risk increased to one in 100,000. (In fact, it may be that *any* "shot" or immunizing stimulus might have done the job of increasing risk, for several cases occurred in people who had received only influenza B vaccine, which shared no antigens with influenza A.)

The critics cried foul again. One scientist even claimed to have predicted that the Guillain-Barré syndrome would be caused by the swine flu vaccine—although the inspiration for that prediction must have been less scientific than mystical, since a careful search of several hundred cases reported in the medical literature yielded only one report of Guillain-Barré syndrome following influenza A immunization, whereas in that same series four had been struck by lightning!

Nonetheless, the program was dead. As of this writing a moratorium still bars the use of swine flu vaccine. Another influenza season will start with the same uncertainty, since the era of the last pandemic strain *is* indeed coming to an end.

Whenever I discuss with scientific friends my role in the story just recounted, they invariably ask what I would recommend if we had it to do over again. The best way I know to answer that question is to describe what happened in the first few days of Legionnaire's disease—that frightening, deadly outbreak of interstitial pneumonia that struck a significant fraction of the members of the American Legion attending a national convention in Philadelphia in the late summer of 1976. The cause of that outbreak took months to decipher and turned out to be a new, previously unrecognized microorganism that was more like a bacterium than a virus, but in the early days of the outbreak when the cluster of respiratory illness and deaths was recognized in Philadelphia, the very real possibility existed that it could be the "swine flu." The kind of pulmonary disease, the ferocity of attack, the apparently common ventilation source of the early sufferers all fitted snugly into a pattern that might have accompanied an outbreak of severe influenza A infection.

The panic that hovered during those first few days was impressive: Even physician friends asked me if I couldn't somehow sneak them a little (still experimental) swine flu vaccine because they had relatives *near* Philadelphia! As I tried then and later to rethink the decision to proceed with the mass immunization program, I kept coming back to the fact that, while Legionnaire's disease turned out to be something else, it *could have been* swine flu. I cannot to this day imagine facing such panic unarmed or with an unmobilized stockpile because the "chances were small" of its happening. We had bought an insurance policy against those chances, and like any other insurance against evil times, I for one was both glad we had it and glad we had not had to collect!

But the epilogue is only half complete, for much else of potential public health significance happened during the 1976–1977 season.

The clamor for public involvement in expert decisions pervaded the vaccine arena as it did many other highly technical areas. Many participants in the movement called consumerism seemed to operate on the assumption that, left to their own devices, the experts would automatically be *wrong*. Mote important, the events surrounding the swine flu campaign had required the intelligent advice and participation of a wide variety of individuals with expertise in fields far from virology who had had to start from "scratch" in understanding the issues. In order to prepare for the future, therefore, Assistant Secretary for Health Cooper initiated a series of events intended to take advantage of lessons bitterly learned. (Dr. Cooper is a man of excellent wit, who, in congratulating NIH's D. Carleton Gadjusek on his new Nobel prize for study of so-called "slow viruses" in November 1976, said rather ruefully that, while he was thrilled at the honor Dr. Gadjusek's recognition reflected on the federal research program in general, he couldn't help hoping that it didn't lead to yet another vaccine!)

First, a National Immunization Conference was assembled in November 1976 on the campus of the National Institutes of Health. Economists, actuaries, lawyers, housewives, ethicists, consumerists, and representatives of volunteer health agencies, and minority groups of all sorts joined the biomedical experts to discuss immunization from the broadest possible point of view. The results as covered by the press were rather strident, for the catchiest phrases, as usual, came from the "radical consumerists"—they used the podium well and their familiar howls against the experts were in full crescendo. In fact, by the third day of the conference their vituperation was so pervasive that it evoked an answering howl from one of the most distinguished, conscientious, and harassed of the "expert advisers" who were their target. Dr. Gene Stollerman, then chairman both of the national group of academic professors of medicine and of the FDA's advisory panel on bacterial vaccines, commented that, to read about the conference and the "expert advisers" in the previous evening's paper, "One would think we were snakes in the grass rather than carriers of the caduceus!" And from Dr. Harry Meyer of the Bureau of Biologics, who for months had been in the center of the whirlwind of accusation, investigation, and litigation, came the marvelous quote (from Jerold Auerbach): "What God spared Egypt, Americans inflict upon themselves."

The conference, then, would have been a disappointment

had the process stopped there, but the effort to broaden the base of public involvement in immunization issues was well-conceived, and Dr. Cooper did not stop with a token conference. The troubles plaguing immunization were obviously serious, and the Office of the Assistant Secretary for Health therefore established working groups to address the urgent questions that had emerged or had been emphasized during the swine flu program. How *should* immunization policy be formulated? What was to be done to ensure continued production and adequate supply of vaccines as the number of companies involved in their manufacture dwindled? Who was liable when rare or unrelated misfortune followed the delivery of a properly manufactured vaccine? (Even as the working group on liability began their task, they knew that the federal office, which was operating under the swine flu legislation to handle claims against the immunization program, had already been buried in an avalanche of suits.) What was the acceptable solution to the seemingly mutually exclusive demands of informed consent versus public health salesmanship: How could you "push" a vaccine while insisting that its recipients sign pages of fine print saying they fully understood that terrible things might befall them in its wake, even when the risks were miniscule? (This was already required for polio vaccine.) And finally, how could you improve the quality of consumer education in immunization so that apathy could be covercome and the public made less vulnerable to fear and confusion introduced by florid journalism during future programs of prevention?

The working groups appointed by Dr. Cooper attacked each of these problems. During the winter when he and Dr. David Sencer, Director of the CDC, became what some called the chief casualties of the swine flu (the Carter administration moved quickly to relieve them both of their duties), the groups with their dozens of members met, argued, and learned from each other.

The result was doubly good: Not only were the hard issues of the 1970s addressed and in many cases met in the reports that emerged; but, perhaps more important, a much broader cadre now had learned and understood the vocabulary and issues of preventive medicine and immunization. To me it was particularly striking, when the groups' recommendations were presented at a Second National Immunization Conference in April of 1977, that the raucous contributions of the "radical consumerists" had been replaced by calm, competent entries from persons who ably articulated the genuine interests and perspectives of the consuming public.

A report of the recommendations of the working groups and the conference was prepared for H.E.W. Secretary Joseph Califano, urging that a National Immunization Commission be established to complement and augment the function of the existing federal expert advisory panels concerning immunization programs. Even as that report was being prepared, however, Secretary Califano—who had not yet appointed a replacement for Dr. Cooper—got a taste of what the trials of the previous year had been. A small outbreak of A/Victoria influenza occurred, and it was suddenly realized that *all* influenza vaccine had been placed under moratorium in the wake of the Guillain-Barré experience. Against a genuine influenza threat, the risk/benefit analysis was very different, and an ad hoc group of advisers was urgently assembled to reconsider and (as it happened) to lift the moratorium, so that the A/Victoria vaccine could be used.

A second crisis arose shortly thereafter; the pharmaceutical manufacturers, as usual, needed six months' lead time to prepare the following year's flu vaccines, and they were awaiting the federal decision as to what strains of influenza would be included in the 1977–1978 formulation. The usual path to such decisions was cluttered with the debris of the previous months' discord, so that Secretary Califano again called an ad hoc group to advise him. This group was constituted to achieve the breadth of expertise and consumer participation said to be lacking in the "swine flu decision," and drew in part on those who had participated in the working groups of the preceding months. The *general* recommendation was reached that the A/Victoria and B/Hong Kong strain prototypes should constitute the new vaccine, and the technical and scientific details were then referred to the preexisting panels of biomedical experts.

Thus, the area of vaccine policy and and decision-making

had undergone a not-so-quiet revolution, and it was evident that things would never be the same again. The casualties of the revolution were numerous; the loss of such distinguished and able public servants as Drs. Cooper and Sencer was a heavy price to pay. Public confidence in vaccines of all sorts had been dangerously eroded, and the astonishing accumulation of litigation in the wake of the swine flu program could only serve to increase the anxieties of the pharmaceutical and insurance industries, leaving them wondering how much further they should venture in the relatively unprofitable business of biologics manufacture. Finally, 75,000,000 doses of swine flu vaccine lay in storage, under moratorium, presumably wasted—unless the experts' 1976 concerns proved to be belatedly justified in the 1977–1978 flu season.

However, the gains, while more difficult to assess at close range, may have been equally significant. Even though the increased visibility of immunization programs was initially achieved through a "bad press," important nonmedical segments of the community had learned of and begun to share the alarm that experts had felt for years at the decreasing levels of immunity among children to polio, measles, diphtheria, and other preventable contagious diseases. Individuals with expertise in virology, immunology, communications arts, law, economics, and industry had been forced to learn each others' vocabulary and then to carry on a conversation about a common problem in the nation's delivery of public health care. Volunteer health agencies had for years felt isolated and excluded from the realm of federally sponsored immunization programs; now, they were at last able to win recognition for their extraordinary expertise at mobilization of public opinion and participation. The scaffolding for a future advisory structure had been designed and then tested; there was room to hope that complex and ominous problems (such as liability) might yet be solved by centering such diverse expertise upon them.

At the end of the Second National Immunization Conference, the bright lights were on again: Secretary Califano arrived to thank the working groups that Assistant Secretary Cooper had initiated months before and to announce another national immunization campaign. This one was to take longer, and the target was different: The battle would be won when at least 90 percent of America's children were protected against polio, measles, diphtheria, tetanus, pertussis, mumps, and rubella. The word "vaccine," which had begun to produce an almost traumatic ring for the experts in the preceding months, sounded good again; and it was a bit astonishing but nonetheless encouraging to see a new, fresh group of enthusiasts enter the arena with flags flying in another campaign of federally sponsored immunization, this one aimed at the very center of the problem: effective preventive medicine.

Appendices

Public Law 94-266, April 15, 1976

Senate Report 94-1147, August 10, 1976

Public Law 94-380 (S. 3735) August 12, 1976

Extract from the Congressional Record,
Volume 122, Number 127, August 26, 1976

Ed. Note: No Senate or House report accompanied the Senate and House passed bill (S. 3735). These Extensions of Remarks, prepared by Congressman Rogers and Lee S. Hyde, M.D., professional staff member of the Committee on Interstate and Foreign Commerce, which were published in the "Congressional Record" on August 26, 1976, fourteen days after the President had signed S. 3735 into law, serve as the House report. (A.J.V.)

Public Law 94-266
94th Congress, H. J. Res. 890
April 15, 1976

Joint Resolution

Making emergency supplemental appropriations for public employment programs, summer youth programs, and preventive health services for the fiscal year ending June 30, 1976, and for other purposes

Resolved by the Senate and House of Representatives of the United States of America in Congress assembled, That the following sums are appropriated, out of any money in the Treasury not otherwise appropriated, for the fiscal year ending June 30, 1976, namely:

Emergency supplemental appropriations, 1976.

TITLE I

INDEPENDENT AGENCIES

ENVIRONMENTAL PROTECTION AGENCY

CONSTRUCTION GRANTS

For an additional amount for liquidation of obligations incurred pursuant to authority contained in section 203 of the Federal Water Pollution Control Act, as amended, $300,000,000, to remain available until expended.

33 USC 1283.

TITLE II

DEPARTMENT OF LABOR

EMPLOYMENT AND TRAINING ADMINISTRATION

COMPREHENSIVE MANPOWER ASSISTANCE

For an additional amount for "Comprehensive manpower assistance", $528,420,000, to remain available until September 30, 1976.

TEMPORARY EMPLOYMENT ASSISTANCE

For expenses necessary to carry out activities authorized by title II of the Comprehensive Employment and Training Act of 1973, as amended (29 U.S.C. 841–851), $1,200,000,000, to remain available until January 31, 1977.

COMMUNITY SERVICE EMPLOYMENT FOR OLDER AMERICANS

To carry out title IX of the Older Americans Act, as amended, $55,900,000, to remain available until June 30, 1977.

42 USC 3056.

90 STAT. 362

DEPARTMENT OF HEALTH, EDUCATION, AND WELFARE

CENTER FOR DISEASE CONTROL

PREVENTIVE HEALTH SERVICES

42 USC 241, 289a.

For an additional amount for "Preventive Health Services" for carrying out, to the extent not otherwise provided, title III and section 431 of the Public Health Service Act for a comprehensive, nationwide influenza immunization program, $135,064,000, to remain available until expended: *Provided*, That vaccines may be supplied to State and local health agencies without charge.

RELATED AGENCY

COMMUNITY SERVICES ADMINISTRATION

COMMUNITY SERVICES PROGRAM

For an additional amount for "Community services program", $23,000,000, to remain available until September 30, 1976.
Approved April 15, 1976.

LEGISLATIVE HISTORY:

HOUSE REPORT No. 94-1004 (Comm. on Appropriations).
SENATE REPORT No. 94-742 (Comm. on Appropriations).
CONGRESSIONAL RECORD, Vol. 122 (1976):
    Apr. 5, considered and passed House.
    Apr. 9, considered and passed Senate, amended.
    Apr. 12, House concurred in Senate amendments.
WEEKLY COMPILATION OF PRESIDENTIAL DOCUMENTS, Vol. 12, No. 16:
    Apr. 15, Presidential statement.

NATIONAL SWINE FLU IMMUNIZATION PROGRAM OF 1976

AUGUST 10, 1976.—Ordered to be printed

Mr. McCLELLAN, from the Committee on Appropriations,
submitted the following

REPORT

[To accompany S. 3735]

The Committee on Appropriations, to which was referred the bill
(S. 3735) to amend the Public Health Service Act to authorize the
establishment and implementation of a national influenza immunization program and to provide an exclusive remedy for persons injured
as a result of inoculation with vaccine under such program reports
the same to the Senate without prejudice or any specific recommendation and presents herewith the following information:

The Appropriations Committee has met and reviewed the programs
and legislative language contained within S. 3735, the proposed
"National Swine Flu Immunization Program of 1976." This legislation was sent to the Senate from the Labor and Public Welfare Committee without a report.

This matter was referred to the Senate Appropriations Committee
on August 10 with instructions to expeditiously report the bill back
to the Senate. The Committee has complied because of the potential
urgency of an immunization program but notes that due to the very
short time constraints imposed, a careful and indepth review was not
possible.

The Committee, however, registers its concern over the possible cost
of this measure and the duplication or conflict in procedures which
have already been established following the enactment of the Emergency Supplemental Appropriations Act which contained $135,064,000
for the Swine Flu program.

Further, this measure sets an entirely new precedent which could
have an adverse impact on other existing and future Federal Immunization programs and on other Federal programs where insurance or
liability costs are not now federally subsidized.

Therefore, the Committee reports this measure back to the Senate
without prejudice or any specific recommendation.

○

57-010

An Act

To amend the Public Health Service Act to authorize the establishment and implementation of an emergency national swine flu immunization program and to provide an exclusive remedy for personal injury or death arising out of the manufacture, distribution, or administration of the swine flu vaccine under such program.

Be it enacted by the Senate and House of Representatives of the United States of America in Congress assembled, That this Act may be cited as the "National Swine Flu Immunization Program of 1976".

National Swine Flu Immunization Program of 1976. 42 USC 201 note.

SEC. 2. Section 317 of the Public Health Service Act (42 U.S.C. 247b) is amended by inserting after subsection (i) the following new subsections:

"(j)(1) The Secretary is authorized to establish, conduct, and support (by grant or contract) needed activities to carry out a national swine flu immunization program until August 1, 1977 (hereinafter in this section referred to as the 'swine flu program'). The swine flu program shall be limited to the following:

"(A) The development of a safe and effective swine flu vaccine.

"(B) The preparation and procurement of such vaccine in sufficient quantities for the immunization of the population of the States.

"(C) The making of grants to State health authorities to assist in meeting their costs in conducting or supporting, or both, programs to administer such vaccine to their populations, and the furnishing to State health authorities of sufficient quantities of such swine flu vaccine for such programs.

Grants.

"(D) The furnishing to Federal health authorities of appropriate quantities of such vaccine.

"(E) The conduct and support of training of personnel for immunization activities described in subparagraphs (C) and (D) of this paragraph and the conduct and support of research on the nature, cause, and effect of the influenza against which the swine flu vaccine is designed to immunize, the nature and effect of such vaccine, immunization against and treatment of such influenza, and the cost and effectiveness of immunization programs against such influenza.

"(F) The development, in consultation with the National Commission for the Protection of Human Subjects of Biomedical and Behavioral Research, and implementation of a written informed consent form and procedures for assuring that the risks and benefits from the swine flu vaccine are fully explained to each individual to whom such vaccine is to be administered. Such consultation shall be completed within two weeks after enactment of this Act, or by September 1, 1976, whichever is sooner. Such procedures shall include the information necessary to advice individuals with respect to their rights and remedies arising out of the administration of such vaccine.

Informed consent form and procedures.

"(G) Such other activities as are necessary to implement the swine flu program.

Reports to
Congress.

"(2) The Secretary shall submit quarterly reports to the Congress on the administration of the swine flu program. Each such report shall provide information on—

"(A) the current supply of the swine flu vaccine to be used in the program;

"(B) the number of persons inoculated with such vaccine since the last report was made under this paragraph and the immune status of the population;

"(C) the amount of funds expended for the swine flu program by the United States, each State, and any other entity participating in the program and the costs of each such participant which are associated with the program, during the period with respect to which the report is made; and

"(D) the epidemiology of influenza in the United States during such period.

Contracts.

"(3) Any contract for procurement by the United States of swine flu vaccine from a manufacturer of such vaccine shall (notwithstanding any other provision of law) be subject to renegotiation to eliminate any profit realized from such procurement (except that with respect to vaccine against the strain of influenza virus known as influenza A/Victoria/75 profit shall be allowed but limited to an amount not exceeding a reasonable profit), as determined pursuant to criteria prescribed by the Secretary, and the contract shall expressly so pro-

Insurance pre-
mium amounts,
refund.

vide. Such criteria shall specify that any insurance premium amount which is included in the price of such procurement contract and which is refunded to the manufacturer under any retrospective, experience-rating plan or similar rating plan shall in turn be refunded to the United States.

"(4) No funds are authorized to be appropriated to carry out the activities of the swine flu program authorized in subparagraphs (A), (B), (D), (E), and (F) of paragraph (1) of this subsection in addi-

Ante, p. 362.
Claims
against the
United States.

tion to the funds appropriated by Public Law 94–266.

"(k)(1)(A) The Congress finds that—

"(i) in order to achieve the participation in the program of the agencies, organizations, and individuals who will manufacture, distribute, and administer the swine flu vaccine purchased and used in the swine flu program and to assure the availability of such vaccine in interstate commerce, it is necessary to protect such agencies, organizations, and individuals against liability for other than their own negligence to persons alleging personal injury or death arising out of the administration of such vaccine;

"(ii) to provide such protection and to establish an orderly procedure for the prompt and equitable handling of claims by persons alleging such injury or death, it is necessary that an exclusive remedy for such claimants be provided against the United States because of its unique role in the initiation, planning, and administration of the swine flu program; and

"(iii) in order to be prepared to meet the potential emergency of a swine flu epidemic, it is necessary that a procedure be instituted for the handling of claims by persons alleging such injury or death until Congress develops a permanent approach for handling claims arising under programs of the Public Health

42 USC 201
note.

Service Act.

"(B) To—
"(i) assure an orderly procedure for the prompt and equitable handling of any claim for personal injury or death arising out of the administration of such vaccine; and
"(ii) achieve the participation in the swine flu program of (I) the manufacturers and distributors of the swine flu vaccine, (II) public and private agencies or organizations that provide inoculations without charge for such vaccine or its administration and in compliance with the informed consent form and procedures requirements prescribed pursuant to subparagraph (F) of paragraph (1) of this subsection, and (III) medical and other health personnel who provide or assist in providing inoculations without charge for such vaccine or its administration and in compliance with such informed consent form and procedures requirements, it is the purpose of this subsection to establish a procedure under which all such claims will be asserted directly against the United States under section 1346(b) of title 28, United States Code, and chapter 171 of such title (relating to tort claims procedure) except as otherwise specifically provided in this subsection.

28 USC 2671 et seq. Liability.

"(2)(A) The United States shall be liable with respect to claims submitted after September 30, 1976 for personal injury or death arising out of the administration of swine flu vaccine under the swine flu program and based upon the act or omission of a program participant in the same manner and to the same extent as the United States would be liable in any other action brought against it under such section 1346(b) and chapter 171, except that—
"(i) the liability of the United States arising out of the act or omission of a program participant may be based on any theory of liability that would govern an action against such program participant under the law of the place where the act or omission occurred, including negligence, strict liability in tort, and breach of warranty;
"(ii) the exceptions specified in section 2680(a) of title 28, United States Code, shall not apply in an action based upon the act or omission of a program participant; and
"(iii) notwithstanding section 2401(b) of title 28, United States Code, if a civil action or proceeding for personal injury or death arising out of the administration of swine flu vaccine under the swine flu program is brought within two years of the date of the administration of such vaccine and is dismissed because the plaintiff in such action or proceeding did not file an administrative claim with respect to such injury or death as required by such chapter 171, the plaintiff in such action or proceeding shall have 30 days from the date of such dismissal or two years from the date the claim arose, whichever is later, in which to file such administrative claim.

Administrative claim, filing deadline.

"(B) For purposes of this subsection, the term 'program participant' as to any particular claim means the manufacturer or distributor of the swine flu vaccine used in an inoculation under the swine flu program, the public or private agency or organization that provided an inoculation under the swine flu program without charge for such vaccine or its administration and in compliance with the

"Program participant."

informed consent form and procedures requirements prescribed pursuant to subparagraph (F) of paragraph (1) of this subsection, and the medical and other health personnel who provided or assisted in providing an inoculation under the swine flu program without charge for such vaccine or its administration and in compliance with such informed consent form and procedures requirements.

"(3) The remedy against the United States prescribed by paragraph (2) of this subsection for personal injury or death arising out of the administration of the swine flu vaccine under the swine flu program shall be exclusive of any other civil action or proceeding for such personal injury or death against any employee of the Government (as defined in section 2671 of title 28, United States Code) or program participant whose act or omission gave raise to the claim.

Attorney General, civil action defense.

"(4) The Attorney General shall defend any civil action or proceeding brought in any court against any employee of the Government (as defined in such section 2671) or program participant (or any liability insurer thereof) based upon a claim alleging personal injury or death arising out of the administration of vaccine under the swine flu program. Any such person against whom such civil action or proceeding is brought shall deliver all process served upon him (or an attested true copy thereof) to whoever is designated by the Secretary to receive such papers, and such person shall promptly furnish copies of the pleadings and process therein to the United States attorney for the district embracing the place wherein the civil action or proceeding is brought, to the Attorney General, and to the Secretary.

"(5)(A) Upon certification by the Attorney General that a civil action or proceeding brought in any court against any employee of the Government (as defined in such section 2671) or program participant is based upon a claim alleging personal injury or death arising out of the administration of vaccine under the swine flu program, such action or proceeding shall be deemed an action against the United States under the provisions of title 28, United States Code, and all references thereto. If such action or proceeding is brought in a district court of the United States, then upon such certification the United States shall be substituted as the party defendant.

"(B) Upon a certification by the Attorney General under subparagraph (A) of this paragraph with respect to a civil action or proceeding commenced in a State court, such action or proceeding shall be removed, without bond at any time before trial, by the Attorney General to the district court of the United States of the district and division embracing the place wherein it is pending and be deemed an action brought against the United States under the provisions of title 28, United States Code, and all references thereto; and the United States shall be substituted as the party defendant. The certification of the Attorney General with respect to program participant status shall conclusively establish such status for purposes of such initial removal. Should a district court of the United States determine on a hearing on a motion to remand held before a trial on the merits that an action or proceeding is not one to which this subsection applies, the case shall be remanded to the State court.

"(C) Where an action or proceeding under this subsection is precluded because of the availability of a remedy through proceedings for compensation or other benefits from the United States as provided by any other law, the action or proceeding shall be dismissed, but in that event the running of any limitation of time for commencing, or filing an application or claim in, such proceedings for compensation or other benefits shall be deemed to have been suspended during the pendency of the civil action or proceeding under this subsection.

"(6) A program participant shall cooperate with the United States in the processing or defense of a claim or suit under such section 1346(b) and chapter 171 based upon alleged acts or omissions of the program participant. Upon the motion of the United States or any other party, the status as a program participant shall be revoked by the district court of the United States upon finding that the program participant has failed to so cooperate, and the court shall substitute such former participant as the party defendant in place of the United States and, upon motion, remand any such suit to the court in which it was instituted.   Cooperation.

28 USC 1346, 2671 et seq.

"(7) Should payment be made by the United States to any claimant bringing a claim under this subsection, either by way of administrative settlement or court judgment, the United States shall have, notwithstanding any provision of State law, the right to recover for that portion of the damages so awarded or paid, as well as any costs of litigation, resulting from the failure of any program participant to carry out any obligation or responsibility assumed by it under a contract with the United States in connection with the program or from any negligent conduct on the part of any program participant in carrying out any obligation or responsibility in connection with the swine flu program. The United States may maintain such action against such program participant in the district court of the United States in which such program participant resides or has its principal place of business.   Payment.

"(8) Within one year of the date of the enactment of the National Swine Flu Immunization Program of 1976, and semiannually thereafter, the Secretary shall submit to the Congress a report on the conduct of settlement and litigation activities under this subsection, specifying the number, value, nature, and status of all claims made thereunder, including the status of claims for recovery made under paragraph (7) of this subsection and a detailed statement of the reasons for not seeking such recovery.   Report to Congress.

"(l) For the purposes of subsections (j) and (k) of this section—   Definitions.

"(1) the phrase 'arising out of the administration' with reference to a claim for personal injury or death under the swine flu program includes a claim with respect to the manufacture or distribution of such vaccine in connection with the provision of an inoculation using such vaccine under the swine flu program;

"(2) the term 'State' includes the District of Columbia, Puerto Rico, the Virgin Islands, Guam, American Samoa, and the Trust Territory of the Pacific Islands; and

"(3) the term 'swine flu vaccine' means the vaccine against the strain of influenza virus known as influenza A/New Jersey/76 (Hsw 1N1), or a combination of such vaccine and the vaccine against the strain of influenza virus known as influenza A/Victoria/75.".

Study.
42 USC 247b
note.

Report to
Congress.

SEC. 3. The Secretary of Health, Education, and Welfare shall conduct, or provide for the conduct of, a study of the scope and extent of liability for personal injuries or death arising out of immunization programs and of alternative approaches to providing protection against such liability (including a compensation system) for such injuries. Within one year of the date of the enactment of this Act, the Secretary shall report to the Congress the findings of such study and such recommendations for legislation (including proposed drafts to carry out such recommendations) as the Secretary deems appropriate.

Approved August 12, 1976.

LEGISLATIVE HISTORY:

SENATE REPORT No. 94-1147 (Comm. on Appropriations).
CONGRESSIONAL RECORD, Vol. 122 (1976):
      Aug. 10, considered and passed Senate and House.
WEEKLY COMPILATION OF PRESIDENTIAL DOCUMENTS, Vol. 12, No. 33:
      Aug. 12, Presidential statement.

Extract from the Congressional Record, Proceedings and Debates of the 94th Congress, Second Session, Volume 122, Number 127, Washington, Thursday, August 26, 1976:

S. 3735—SWINE FLU PROGRAM

Speech of Hon. Paul G. Rogers of Florida in the House of Representatives, Tuesday, August 10, 1976

Mr. ROGERS. Mr. Speaker, I rise again in support of S. 3735. I think before concluding the debate that I should ask the indulgence of my colleagues and take a few minutes to summarize the legislation before us, make some comments on its possible costs, give a general history, explanation, and finally go through a section-by-section analysis of the provisions of the proposal.

SUMMARY OF 3735
NATIONAL SWINE FLU IMMUNIZATION PROGRAM
OF 1976

S. 3735 amends the present Public Health Service Act provisions in section 317 relating to vaccination and other disease control programs to authorize the Secretary of HEW to establish, conduct, and support needed activities to carry out a national swine flu immunization program until August 1, 1977.

The immunization program is to consist of: First, the development of a safe and effective vaccine against the swine flu; second, the preparation and procurement of such vaccine in sufficient quantities for the immunization of the population of the States; third, the making of grants to State health authorities to assist in meeting their costs in conducting or supporting, or both, immunization programs for State residents and the furnishing of sufficient quantities of the vaccine for such programs; fourth the furnishing to Federal health authorities of appropriate quantities of the vaccine; fifth the conduct and support of training of personnel for the immunization programs as well as the conduct and support of research on the nature, cause and effect of swine flu, the nature and effect of the vaccine, immunization against and treatment of the swine flu, and the cost and effectiveness of the immunization programs; and sixth the development, in consultation with the National Commission for the Protection of Human Subjects of Biomedical Research, and implementation of a written informed consent notice and procedures for assuring that the risks and benefits from the swine flu vaccine are fully explained to each individual to whom the vaccine is to be administered. This form is to be available within 2 weeks of enactment of the bill, or September 1, 1976, whichever is sooner, and is to include the information necessary to advise persons with respect to their rights and remedies arising out of the administration of the vaccine.

The Secretary of HEW is to provide a quarterly report on the administration of the program including a report on the current supply of vaccine, the number of persons inoculated, the amount of funds expended by the United States and any other entities for the program, and the epidemiology of influenza in the United States during the reporting period.

Any contract for procurement by the United States of swine flu vaccine is to be subject to renegotiation to eliminate any profit realized from such procurement, except that a reasonable profit may be allowed for vaccines against the currently prevalent strain of influenza known as A/Victoria/75.

The legislation contains congressional findings on the necessity of establishing a procedure for the making of liability claims against the United States if the vaccination program is to succeed, and provides that the Federal Government will be liable with respect to any claims submitted after September 30, 1976, for personal injury or death resulting from the administration of vaccine under the program based upon the act or omission of a "program participant." An action will be allowed against the Federal Government if it could otherwise have been brought against a private individual under the law of the place where the act or omission occurred.

A "program participant" means the manufacturer or distributor of the swine flu vaccine used in an inoculation in the program, the public or private agencies or organizations that provide an inoculation under the program without charge for the vaccine or its administration and in compliance with the informed consent requirements, and the medical or other personnel who provided or assisted in providing an inoculation under the program without charge for the vaccine or its administration and in compliance with the informed consent requirements.

The remedy against the Federal Government provided is to be the exclusive remedy available to individuals claiming injury or death due to administration of the vaccine. Procedures for carrying out such suits and for their defense by the Attorney General are set out in the bill, and generally follow those of the Federal Tort Claims Act. Should payment be made by the United States to any claimant under the authority, whether by administrative settlement or court judgment, the Federal Government will have the right to recover that portion of the damages paid, as well as any costs of litigation, resulting from the failure of any program participant to carry out any obligation or responsibility assumed by it under a contract with the Federal Government in connection with the program or from any negligent conduct on the part of any program participant in carrying out any obligation or responsibility in connection with the swine flu program.

Within 1 year of enactment, and semiannually thereafter, the Secretary is to submit to Congress a report on the conduct of settlement and litigation activities under the authority to sue the United States specifying the number, value, nature and status of all claims made against the Government and by it for recovery of damages. A detailed statement of the reasons for not seeking recovery of damages paid by the Government, when not sought, must also be provided.

The Secretary is to conduct a study of the scope and extent of liability for personal injuries or deaths arising out of immunization programs and of alternative approaches—including a compensation system—to providing protection against such liability for such injuries. The Secretary is to report within 1 year of enactment on the results of the study and any recommendations for legislation.

COST OF LEGISLATION

The cost of the proposal has been estimated by the Congressional Budget Office in the following cost estimate. It should be noted that the principal cost of the program, the $135 million of Federal funds appropriated previously by Public Law 94-266, is not included in the estimate because it has already been appropriated. Additional appropriations are possible under the legislation, see the section-by-section analysis, but are not specified in the proposed legislation and, therefore, are not estimated. Were additional appropriations made, they would principally be for the costs of State and local programs not covered by the $135 million and these costs would be unlikely to exceed another $25 to $30 million. The Congressional Budget Office estimate is for the expenses likely to be experienced by the Federal Government in the handling of liability claims under the proposed legislation and makes a reasonable set of assumptions to arrive at the estimate in the absence of any more definitive way of establishing the cost.

The total potential cost, $135 million already appropriated plus $7.7 million for handling claims, seems an entirely reasonable investment when compared to the $4 billion in economic costs experienced by the United States during the most recent, and mildest of the influenza epidemics which this country has experienced. This was the epidemic of the Hong Kong strain of influenza in 1968 which produced approximately 30,000 excess deaths in the United States.

I include the following:

CONGRESSIONAL BUDGET OFFICE: COST ESTIMATE

1. Bill number: S. 3735.
2. Bill title: National Influenza Program of 1976.
3. Purpose of bill: Authorizes the Secretary of the Department of Health, Education, and Welfare to conduct a national program of immunization against the strain of influenza caused by the virus A/New Jersey/76 (Hsw 1/N/1) (commonly known as swine flu) and to make the federal government liable, under the Federal Torts Claim Act, for all claims in connection with injuries resulting from the inoculation program. The bill also authorizes the government to seek recovery of claims

paid by the government from third parties (drug manufacturers, providers, etc.) where negligence can be attributed to those third parties.

4. Cost estimate: ($ in millions).

	1977	1978	1979	1980	1981	Total
Liability payments...............	.51	2.58	2.06	—	—	5.15
Administrative costs............	1.29	3.23	.65	—	—	5.17
Recovery from third parties	—	—	-.65	-1.29	-.64	-2.58
Total............................	1.80	5.81	2.06	-1.29	-.64	7.74

5. Basis for estimate: Much of the data utilized in this estimate is based upon work done by the actuaries at the Federal Insurance Administration (FIA) although, in some cases, modified by the Congressional Budget Office (CBO). The actuaries projected that actual injury would occur in one case per million inoculations (based on a projected 172 million inoculations). CBO has increased this ratio to 2 per million because of the rapidity with which this program will be implemented and the large volume of vaccines to be produced and used. Also, FIA has projected the ratio of claims filed to claims awarded to be between 10 and 100 to 1. For the purpose of this estimate, a ratio of 50 to 1 was used. Thus, based upon the projected 344 cases where an award would be made and the 50 to 1 ratio, a total of 17,200 claims would be filed. FIA further assumed, based on a malpractice claims study in Florida, that 50 percent of the claims filed would require significant processing time. Actual costs for liability and claims litigation were calculated using the above assumptions and an average benefit payment of $15,000 (based on a nationwide average payment for a malpractice claim) and an administrative cost of $600 per claim) this was determined by utilizing the experience of the VA in processing malpractice claims).

To determine the yearly costs, it was assumed that 50 percent of the claims would be filed during the first year, but half the litigation of those claims would extend into 1978. It was further assumed that the rest of the claims would be filed in 1978, but 25 percent of the processing time needed for those claims would extend into 1979. With regard to liability, 10 percent of the payments are assumed in 1977, 50 percent in 1978, and 40 percent in 1979.

Lastly, recovery from third parties is assumed in 50 percent of the cases, with 25 percent of that amount recovered in 1979, 50 percent in 1980, and 25 percent in 1981.

6. Estimate comparison: Not Applicable.

7. Previous CBO estimate: None.

8. Estimate prepared by Jeffrey C. Merrill (225-4972).

9. Estimate approved by: James L. Blum, Assistant Director for Budget Analysis.

HISTORY, EXPLANATION, AND JUSTIFICATION OF THE PROPOSED LEGISLATION

INFLUENZA

Understanding the need for the National Swine Flu Immunization program and, therefore, the proposed legislation, S. 3735, requires first an understanding of influenza. Influenza is a highly contagious acute disease caused by one of the several types of the influenza virus. It has a short 1- to 3-day incubation period and is characterized by sudden onset with fever, prostration, generalized aches and pains—usually in the back and legs—headache, weakness, and loss of appetite. In the respiratory system symptoms are usually mild and "cold" like. This is part of the reason that many people confuse the common cold with influenza leading to a common impression that influenza is more common than is in fact the case. It is, nevertheless, a common disease and those who have had a real case can usually recognize the difference between it and a cold. Influenza lasts 2 to 5 days—although the weakness may persist for some time afterwards. It is rarely fatal but can cause death either acutely, with overwhelming untreatable virus pneumonia within the first few days of illness, or secondarily with a bacterial pneumonia which follows the viral disease and is treatable. Influenza is most dangerous for high risk groups such as the very old, the very young, the debilitated with chronic diseases, and people receiving treatment for diseases such as cancer which suppresses their normal defense mechanisms.

Influenza may be sporadic or epidemic. Epidemics occur every 1 to 4 years and follow minor mutations or changes in the virus which make some people who are immune to the disease susceptible again. During last fall and winter the United States experienced one such "routine" epidemic from the Victoria strain of the virus. Approximately every 10 years the virus undergoes a major mutation and these major new strains usually become epidemic throughout the world, or pandemic. Thus, there were pandemics of Puerto Rican influenza in 1943-44, Asian influenza in 1957-58, and Hong Kong influenza in 1968-69. The new strains are normally named after the area in which they are first identified. The magnitude of these pandemics is measured by the number of excess deaths which occur during the epidemic because of the influenza in excess of the expected number of deaths when influenza is not present. The 1957-58 Asian flu epidemic by this measure caused 80,000 excess deaths and the milder 1968-69 Hong Kong influenza caused 33,000 excess deaths.

Influenza is now the only disease which has the capacity to close schools and places of work because of the number of people who may be felled by it simultaneously in a given community during an epidemic. It is also the only remaining disease which regularly produces any excess deaths which are not compensated by a subsequent decrease in the normal mortality curve. The disease is this important because, while nearly everybody who gets it survives, such a large number of people get it that the small proportion who die may still be a large absolute number.

Economists have attempted to measure the cost of pandemics of influenza by placing dollar values on the medical care required by the victims, the amount of time they lose from work, and similar effects of the epidemic. By this approach the mildest recent pandemic, that of Hong Kong flu in 1968-69, had an economic cost to the United States of $3.9 billion.

SWINE AND SPANISH INFLUENZA

In early January at Fort Dix, N.J., the State of New Jersey cultured for the first time from normal people a new major strain of influenza.

Subsequent studies of soldiers at Fort Dix reported that 1 soldier died, the virus was grown from 12 other soldiers with flu, and approximately 500 had apparently had subclinical cases because their body defense mechanisms demonstrated a response to the disease. Thus, what happened at Fort Dix can be character-ized as a small, self-contained outbreak of a new major strain of influenza in which human-to-human spread occurred but, fortunately, was not sustained. The new flu is called swine flu because it is also found in pigs, although it is not normally caught from associating with pigs or by eating pork.

This new strain caused infected people to develop antibodies—part of the body's defense mechanism—which are identical to those that people developed to the influenza which caused the world-wide pandemic in 1918–19 that resulted in approximately 450,000 deaths in the United States and between 20 and 30 million deaths worldwide. The new flu cannot be said to be the same as the Spanish influenza which caused the 1918–19 epidemic because the virus which caused that epidemic is not available, but there is some evidence that major strains do recur. Thus, the 1958 Asian flu produced the same antibody reactions as did the flu virus which caused the pandemic in 1890.

While the new strain bears some resemblance to the Spanish flu, nobody can say whether or not it would be as devastating as that one since its identification with it is only partial.

However, it should be emphasized that any similarity to the influenza experienced in 1918–19 is disturbing since it was unique in several respects. First, it killed a substantially higher percentage of those it infected than normal. Second, it killed a remarkable number of healthy young adults with an acute overwhelming virus pneumonia that, it must be emphasized, would still not always be treatable in 1976 because viruses are not killed by antibiotics and the pneumonia was so acute and so severe that it would not always be treatable with respirators. Third, the disease had such high attack rates and swept both the whole country and any given community so fast that there was no way to control it or plan for it once it arrived. Thus, it overwhelmed the available hospital and medical resources, killing as many as 700 people in a single day in Philadelphia. The unusual "W-shaped" mortality curve of the 1918–19 epidemic is shown in figure 1 and the rapid spread of the epidemic in figure 2. These figures are adapted from Alfred W. Crosby's excellent history of the 1918–19 epidemic, "Epidemic and Peace, 1918," published this year. The fast spread is not unusual; when the Victoria strain appeared in this country this year it was subsequently identified in 47 States in less than 2 months.

It must be understood that the proposed influenza immunization program can be justified entirely by comparing its costs to those of the mildest epidemic of influenza which this country experienced, that of Hong Kong flu in 1968–69. By this comparison the effort described in the remainder of these remarks is entirely justifiable on a cost-benefit basis without reference to what happened in 1918–19. However, the similarity is noteworthy and disturbing.

The debate over the swine flu program was complicated in late July and early August by the appearance of the infamous legion fever in Pennsylvania. To the enormous relief of all involved this did not prove to be swine flu, although the case of this mysterious and dangerous fever is still unknown, and did not spread beyond those initially affected. What was disturbing was the remarkable resemblance between the onset and course of legion fever, characterized as it was by an overwhelming untreatable pneumonia, and the descriptions of the severe cases of influenza experienced by young adults in 1918. Further study, and discovery of the cause of legion fever, is awaited with interest in hopes that any further outbreaks can be prevented. In the meantime the need to protect the population against the possible outbreak of swine flu remains as real as it would be if legion fever had never appeared, albeit perhaps a little easier to understand.

THE PROPOSED NATIONAL IMMUNIZATION PROGRAM

The "normal" appearance of a major new strain of the flu involves sporadic outbreaks of the new strain in the spring and summer of the year in which it is first identified and the development of a full pandemic in the fall and winter of that year. This normal pattern and the identification of an outbreak at Ft. Dix clearly support the conclusion that it is possible, although nobody knows what the chances are, that the local outbreak at Ft. Dix will lead to a major epidemic in the fall. Since the Ft. Dix episode, extensive efforts have been made on the part of the Center

for Disease Control and the rest of the world's disease surveillance
network to identify subsequent cases of the swine flu. Despite
rumors of such cases in Australia and the Philippines, none have
yet been identified, except for a very small number of individual
cases in people who each had a history of exposure to pigs and
were under treatment for cancer. A new outbreak would certainly
increase the unknown chances that an epidemic of the new virus
will occur in the fall or winter. Equally, as time passes without
identifying such outbreaks the chances diminish. However, it is
not safe to say that the epidemic will not occur at least until after
the coming flu season, and while the odds may be slim they must
be considered real and the enormous potential costs of an epidemic remembered.

Given the possibility of an epidemic, HEW officials and
national experts on influenza recommended in March that President Ford initiate a massive campaign for the immediate development of a vaccine against the new flu strain and the production of
enough of the vaccine to immunize the entire U.S. population.
President Ford proposed such a program and sought appropriation of the necessary funds by the Congress by the first of April in
the amount of $135 million. Such an effort has not been made
previously because there has not been an adequate warning of a
possible epidemic before. Some attempt was made with Hong
Kong flu in 1968 but once recognized it reappeared and spread too
rapidly.

The Subcommittee on Health and the Environment held
hearings on the President's proposal on March 31, 1976. At that
time witnesses were heard from HEW, vaccine manufacturers,
State and local health officials, representatives of major provider
organizations including the American Public Health Association,
the American Medical Association and the American Hospital
Association, and the Health Research Group. All witnesses before
the committee agreed with the President's proposal and urged its
immediate pursuit with the exception of the Health Research
Group which expressed caution and recommended consideration
of immunizing solely the high risk population. While charges
were heard that the proposal might have been politically moti-

vated, the subcommittee concluded that whether or not this was the case it was nevertheless a correct proposal and proceeded to recommend legislation authorizing the program.

The $135 million was appropriated by Public Law 94-226, signed April 15, and is being used for the purchase of the vaccine, Federal grants to the States to meet their costs of operating the necessary mass immunization programs, and for Federal costs of regulating the development of the new vaccine and doing related research. The original estimate of the cost of purchasing the vaccine was $100 million at 50 cents a dose for 200 million people. It is currently hoped that the cost will not reach this total cost since the preliminary indications are that the vaccine is being made for as little as 20 cents to 30 cents a dose, the full 200 million doses may not be needed if some people choose not to receive the vaccine, and the proposed legislation should reduce the costs of insurance for the manufacturers—which it must be assumed will be included in the price of the vaccine. It is clear at this point that the original estimate of $26 million for grants to State health departments for their costs was inadequate and any funds not spent on the purchase of vaccine should be made available to States. Further, consideration should be given, if they can demonstrate their additional costs, to the appropriation of additional funds to meet them.

THE VACCINE

Since the appropriation, approximately 100 million doses of vaccine have been produced by the four manufacturers of influenza vaccines. While essentially similar to previous vaccines which have been in extensive use among millions of people since 1940, the new vaccine has been subject to more extensive clinical trial than any previous flu vaccine and has proven itself both remarkably safe and remarkably effective in adults over age 24. Thus, in this group some 70 to 95 percent of recipients had antibody responses which would protect them against infection for at least a year. No severe side effects were experienced and only 1.9 percent experienced mild side effects such as a sore arm, transient low grade fever, or headache. This number compares with the 1.7 percent of those who received a placebo injection of salt water who experienced similar side effects.

This experience is not surprising. The influenza vaccine is a killed virus vaccine made from viruses grown in fertile chicken eggs. Since the virus is killed it cannot produce an actual case of influenza. While the vaccine still carries a reputation as one which can cause bad reactions, this reputation has not been deserved since new centrifugation technology made successful separation of the virus from egg constituents possible. Nevertheless, people with a history of egg allergy will be warned of the possibility of an allergic reaction and should probably not take the vaccine.

The protection from influenza vaccine lasts for only a year or two at most. Thus, it will be important to ascertain whether successful protection of the population against an epidemic this fall which occurred in the rest of the world during the subsequent year would have to be repeated later so that the effect is not merely to delay the epidemic. This is important because efforts to immunize the United States population would probably not succeed in protecting the rest of the world against the flu epidemic if it is going to occur. This is because influenza is so highly contagious that "herd" immunity is hard to achieve even in a population with high rates of immunization. Thus, cases could still occur and would be likely to spread, although those who had received the vaccine would be protected.

The United States is apparently the only country with the capacity to contemplate successful immunization of the whole population and at this point is the only country undertaking the proposed program. The World Health Organization in reviewing this situation indicated its agreement with the U.S. effort although medical literature in other countries has expressed concern that the odds of an epidemic may not be worth the cost and effort.

There has been much discussion of use of the flu vaccine in people under 24 because, while the vaccine is effective in producing immunity to influenza in all ages, the rate at which side effects are experienced increases as the age of the recipient decreases. This is why it is not normally recommended for children and why to date HEW researchers have been unable to recommend a dosage for people under 18. Those who have received it who are under 18 have been protected but have experienced slightly higher, presently unacceptable rates of side effects than those over 18. HEW is continuing to do research in the young population designed to establish a dose or schedule of doses which will provide protection without excessive side effects. They have offered every assurance that they will not recommend that children of any age receive vaccine until a safe and effective dose has been established. Further, the plan is to work down gradually in age groups so that for instance a dose is established for children over 6 before it is attempted for children under 6. This cautious approach seems reasonable and properly reflects the fact that people under 20 are generally not at very high risk of death from influenza.

IMPLEMENTATION OF THE PROGRAM

While the manufacture and testing of the vaccine have gone forward, HEW and the States have engaged in extensive preparation for delivering it upon its purchase by the Federal Government. The general strategy will be for the States to receive the vaccine from the Federal Government and then provide it with some funds to city and county health departments. Twenty to 40 million doses of a bivalent vaccine protecting against both swine and Victoria flu will be available for the usual high risk population. The health departments, in cooperation with other agencies and the help of volunteer professionals, will conduct mass immunization programs of the type previously used for polio vaccine in Sabin Oral Sunday programs, and measles and rubella vaccine programs in past years. These programs will be held in schools, health departments, churches, places of business and other locations easily accessible to large populations on advertised dates. Each person seeking the immunization will be given a statement of the risks and benefits and asked to give his informed consent to receipt of the vaccine. Records will be kept of who received which vaccine and of the consent. Some vaccine will be made available to physicians and hospitals for their use in supplying their own patients. The details are going to vary from State to State at the State's discretion and no State, other program participant or potential recipient is being required to participate.

HEW is also responsible for some public awareness efforts—a clearly deficient part of the program to date—and related documentation and research. To date the needed biomedical and epidemiological research and surveillance activities have been satisfactory. Needed operational and health services research is not being sufficiently pursued although it is authorized by the legislation.

Substantial attention has been devoted to how the program is to be paid for and whether or not it is to involve profit. Because the bulk of the costs and responsibility are being undertaken by Federal, State, and local government it has been felt by many that the vaccine should be available to people without charge and that those who participate in the program should not make profit from it. This concern has received particular attention since the various participants have discovered the need for the proposed special legislation which will protect them in some degree from the normal risks of doing business. For these reasons the proposed legislation goes beyond requirements already imposed by HEW that people not be charged for the actual cost of the vaccine and requires in addition that people not be charged for the administrative cost of supplying them with the vaccine.

Thus, the protection from liability in the first instance offered by the legislation is available only to those who give the vaccine with no charge of any kind to the recipient. Further, the legislation requires that the vaccine be made available by the manufacturers without profit. In this connection it is reassuring that all four of the manufacturers of the vaccine have indicated their willingness to do this given the special nature of the program and the required legislation. An exception has been provided for the A/Victoria vaccine, already made by the manufacturers in anticipation of normal market profit, when it is purchased by the Federal Government for inclusion in bivalent vaccine to be given to the high risk population.

Several substantial concerns with respect to the developing

programs have been expressed. Adequate efforts have clearly not been made to interpret and advertise the program to the public which may mean participation in it will be low. The various logistical and supply problems involved may not be met within the time frame contemplated. There is concern about the damage which participation in the program may cause ongoing activities of State and local health departments whose resources must be committed to the program. In large degree it is hoped that the latter problem can be solved through the use of volunteers and temporary employment under such programs as the CETA program. However, in general, the designed program appears both warranted and reasonably well underway. In addition, the proposed legislation gives sufficient authority to solve all these problems if it is used effectively by HEW.

LIABILITY

The real problem has not been with either the scientific decision to have a program or its implementation, but with the risk of suits by people who sustain—or feel they have sustained—injury from receiving the vaccine and with the need for insurance against that risk of suit. In early June all four of the manufacturers of the vaccine experienced either cancellation or limitation of their liability insurance for costs of claims handling, legal fees and damages in connection with their liability for injuries sustained by those who receive the vaccine. The manufacturers all then threatened not to sell the vaccine without insurance. This prompted HEW to try in the contract for purchase of the vaccine to assume some of the risks of such possible damages in hopes that this would make adequate insurance available in the private sector for whatever residual risk remained with the manufacturers. HEW was prevented from doing so by the Anti-Deficiency Act of 1921 which precludes Government agencies from incurring obligations in advance of appropriations without specific authority for doing so. HEW then proposed legislation (H.R. 14409 and H.R. 14437) which would have authorized assumption of the risk by permitting indemnification of the manufacturers when they suffered certain losses for some reasons.

Since that time it has been made amply clear by representatives of the insurance industry that, without some form and degree of assumption of the legal risks of the program by the Federal Government, they would not insure the manufacturers for the program. In addition to the collapse of the insurance market for liability for the manufacturers, the subcommittee also became aware during June and July of growing evidence that the market might collapse more generally for liability and malpractice insurance for other participants in the program. Thus, the State of Washington was given an estimate for coverage of $3 million—approximately $1 a shot—and San Mateo County, Calif., received an estimate for insurance for its participation in the program from its insurer—the California Hospital Association—of $1.76 per shot or $800,000. These estimates were given as redeterminations of the premium for the insurance coverage already available if the agency participated in the program. The justification was that each immunization would be an outpatient visit, that the program would create a substantial change in the number of outpatient visits experienced by the agency under its insurance coverage, and that therefore the premium for that coverage should be adjusted. Other insurers of participants in the program began to consider reinsuring their insurance, another sign of change and instability in the insurance market when it has not previously been done. These growing indications of collapse of the market for insurance for liability, coupled with clear indications that people would not participate in the program without such insurance, finally led the subcommittee to include all participants in the program in the proposed legislation rather than just the vaccine manufacturers, although the manufacturers were the first ones to experience difficulty.

The special problems of the manufacturers arose out of recent cases (*Davis* v. *Wyeth Laboratories, Inc.*, 339 F. 2d 121 (9th Circuit 1968) and *Reyes* v. *Wyeth Laboratories, Inc.*, 498 F. 2d 1264 (5th Circuit 1974)) in which the manufacturers of Sabin oral polio vaccine were held liable to the plaintiffs who were found to have contracted polio from the vaccine even though the plaintiffs did not establish negligence in the manufacture of the vaccine. In both cases the courts applied the "strict products liability" rule set forth in section 402(A) of the Restatement—Second—of Torts of 1965 in which the manufacturer of a so-called unavoidably unsafe product has a duty to see to it that proper warning of the hazards of the use of the product reach the user. These cases make it possible that the manufacturers could be held liable for injuries for which they had no negligent responsibility in the ordinary sense of the word because the person involved failed to receive a warning of some risk of the vaccine. While the risks of this occurring seem remote given that the cases apply to live vaccines and influenza vaccine is a killed vaccine and given the direct contractual assumption of the duty to warn proposed by the HEW, the approximate measure of the risk which would have to be assumed by the Federal Government in order to make insurance by the private sector possible was the risks associated with the responsibilities being assumed by the Government including the duty to warn.

It must be underlined that it has never been clear to the subcommittee what the fuss has all been about. The four vaccine manufacturers during the last 5 years have produced over 70 million doses of flu vaccine which has been received by the high risk population and have produced fewer than 20 claims against them. The vaccine is a killed vaccine and clearly both safe and effective. The department's proposals for obtaining informed consent from those who receive the vaccine seemed at least adequate. Thus at least some Members clearly felt the manufacturers and insurers were faint-hearted, shirking their social responsibilities, or unreasonably pursuing profit or precedent. However, vigorous pursuit of the issue throughout the months of June and July made it clear that, whatever the merits of the situation, a program was not possible without insurance and that insurance was not going to be available without legislation.

It further became clear that the delay resulting from the situation was finally in late July beginning to delay the implementation of the program. This delay arose when the manufacturers, who had through the end of June and into July been making vaccine without assurance of any contract for its purchase, began in late July to gradually curtail production after making close to 100 million doses. Curtailed production delays the program longer than the period of indecision because it takes disproportionate amounts of time to gear production up again once it is stopped. Thus, the subcommittee found itself in the unpleasant situation of having to make a decision as to whether or not a program was necessary and enact legislation to break the impasse in as expeditious a manner as possible.

For this reason it was made entirely clear that the approach finally chosen is not necessarily the best one to use in other situations, if they should occur, that the proposed legislation is not intended to suggest any precedent for the future with respect to the problems considered during the debate, and that it certainly leaves some details to be resolved by HEW. However, the program was judged necessary in view of the possible costs and benefits and therefore the legislation provided.

Further, it seemed to many in the debate that the issues being raised are not going to be one time issues and that therefore they will require further study and consideration. For this reason, the proposed legislation contains requirements that these studies be undertaken by HEW and provided to the committee within a year. Possible precedents which were evidently of concern to the various parties during the debate were the possibility that participants in the program would make either any or unreasonable profit from it, that the vaccine manufacturers would relieve themselves of liabilities to which they should still be held, that the vaccine manufacturers would begin to place responsibility for the production of unprofitable drugs in the public sector while retaining the right to manufacture the profitable drugs, or that the insurance industry would similarly succeed in avoiding any responsibility for providing insurance in risky or unprofitable situations—presumably leaving this responsibility with the Government—while continuing to retain the right to write insurance in safe and profitable situations.

The largest and most important issue in the debate has clearly been liability and malpractice insurance. Liability insurance for many years has been part of a system of social insurance which this society uses to provide compensation for people who are injured by products and services which they obtain from the marketplace. Under this system people who are injured sue those from whom they receive the product or service, and, if the court finds that they suffered injuries because of some negligence on the part of the provider, they receive financial compensation for the injury. Providers of goods and services plan for such settlements by buying insurance against them and including the cost of the insurance in the price of the product or service. Thus, most people buy a form of insurance against injury from the product when they buy the product. To date a key concept in this system has been its limitation to injury in negligence situations; it is a fault system. Only in workmen's and unemployment compensation, and no-fault auto insurance systems have social insurance programs for injury been created which do not require finding of fault to function. Evidence of problems with this scheme of tort liability and insurance against it has been growing in recent years and can be found in the debate over no-fault auto insurance, the malpractice crisis, and such parochial matters for the Subcommittee on Health and the Environment as the availability of liability insurance for the PSRO program.

The subcommittee to date would take no position on the source of these troubles or their possible solutions. They clearly arise in situations in which the quality of services are poorly policed, from the litigious quality of the era, from increased public insistence on its rights, and a host of other factors. Nor is it possible now to anticipate correct solutions. However, there is growing indication that at least with respect to public immunization programs this is not likely to prove an unusual situation. Thus, other countries have already found it necessary to enact special legislation dealing with these problems—most of which take a no-fault patient compensation approach, like that already in use in Sweden, see Cohen and Korper, "The Swedish No-Fault Patient Compensation Program," in the Insurance Law Journal, 637: 70–80, 2/76—and HEW has begun to experience difficulties with routine purchase of vaccine for ongoing public immunization programs in connection with these issues.

It should be noted in this connection that, to the extent that negligence, strict liability and breach of warranty remain at issue, they need definition. They are clearly terms which have taken on special meanings in the legal debate and these need to be defined and agreed upon. This is thus one of the tasks which it is hoped that the Department will undertake in the studies required by this legislation. It seemed unclear to some parties to the debate, for instance, whether or not the concept of negligence has already been extended by courts to allow the tort liability system to function in situations in which injuries occur without any negligence in the ordinary sense on the part of any party, such as reactions to immunizations properly given, allergie reactions (see Yarborough's "Strict Liability and Allergic Drug Reactions," *Mississippi Law Journal*, 47:526-43, 1976), or injuries sustained in the course of human experimentation. Much of the difficulty of this debate has been caused by lack of clear understanding and agreement about who is, and should be, responsible for compensating injuries in various possible situations. The distinctions and responsibilities intended in the proposed legislation are described in the section-by-section analysis of subsection 317(k) (4).

POSSIBLE SOLUTIONS

The approach originally chosen by HEW to the problem of the risk of liability arising out of the program was to authorize the government to indemnify the manufacturers for losses arising out of inoculation of the vaccine except when the losses arose from failure of the manufacturer to exercise due care in the manufacture or handling of the vaccine in accordance with the contract specifications or for failure to discharge properly any other obligation under the contract. This approach is only one of several possible options which were considered by the subcommittee. The Government could have proposed to reinsure in some degree insurance companies which provided insurance to the manufacturers for the risks, as has been done in flood, riot, and nuclear energy catastrophe insurance programs. Either of these two approaches could have been offered to other participants in the program besides the vaccine manufacturers, although in their cases to do so only for non-negligent losses after they were incurred would not have been as helpful. These alternatives were ultimately rejected because they could only be used if the private market would function with them and no assurance of this was available, they did not offer any hope of controlling profits or costs, and they did not solve the real problem of other program participants—baseless suits.

Other alternatives were available, including the one used in the proposed legislation—and therefore described and discussed more extensively in the rest of these remarks—and the possibility of creating a program for direct compensation of patients injured by the vaccine, similar to workmen's compensation programs, which would have precluded suits in connection with the program, and provided for administrative determination of compensation amounts for medical and economic losses suffered by the injured. Many parties to the debate felt that this solution was conceptually perhaps the best but that it would prove more controversial than the use of the tort claims approach that was chosen and would not be implementable by HEW within the available time. Since such an approach has been used successfully in other countries, been recommended by legal scholars in this country (see Smith's *Liability in Preventive Medicine*, June 1973, Baynes' *Liability for Vaccine Related Injuries*, January 1975, and the work of Curran and Pies, and Ladimer, and Havighurst and Tancredi) and has precedent in situations like workmen's compensation programs, it seemed clear that it could work and would be constitutional. It, thus, should certainly be included in the approaches studied and described in the studies mandated by the legislation.

THE SEARCH FOR A SOLUTION

The original HEW proposal for partial assumption by the Federal Government of liability arising out of the program via indemnification of the vaccine manufacturers for losses, absent negligence on their part, was extensively debated and considered by the Subcommittee on Health and the Environment during the months of June and July. It required, as a condition of its success, that the normal insurance market function in support of the program and primary emphasis was given by the subcommittee to trying to assure that this would be the case. The subcommittee held hearings on June 28 on the original legislative proposal and at these hearings representatives were heard from HEW, the vaccine manufacturers, State and local health officials, Doctors Jonas Salk and Albert Sabin, and the Health Research Group. At this time continued support for the program was voiced by all witnesses except for Dr. Sabin and the Health Research Group who both agreed that the high risk population should be immunized but were not convinced that the attempt to immunize the entire population should be pursued.

Dr. Sabin suggested that the vaccine should be stockpiled and delivered only at such time as the influenza reappeared. This proposal, while reasonable on its face, seemed unlikely to protect the population against an epidemic if the virus reappeared because it would take at least several weeks, if not a month or two, to deliver the vaccine and even after people receive the vaccine they would need an additional 2 to 4 weeks to develop immunity to the disease. This time lapse would, from previous experience with the spread of influenza epidemics, offer no assurance that people would be protected against the disease before they were exposed to it, since it is known that it can spread through the entire country within 4 to 6 weeks.

After the hearings on the 28th of June the subcommittee requested that the vaccine manufacturers and HEW continue their contract negotiations in hopes of arriving at a satisfactory contract, either without legislation or with a clear understanding of what legislation would be necessary and what the terms of the contract which the legislation would make possible would be. Further hearings were held on July 20 at which time HEW reported that they had been unable to obtain satisfactory contract terms or any assurance that, if a contract could be written, the manufacturers would be insured for their participation in the program.

The subcommittee then held further hearings on July 23 at

which it heard from the chief executive officers of some 15 major insurance companies and succeeded in extracting a commitment from them that they would try to write a pool of insurance on the program. This was offered despite their belief that the program was uninsurable in the traditional sense because they had no basis on which to estimate the risks, anticipated numerous nuisance suits which would nevertheless have to be defended by their legal staffs, had experienced extensive losses in products liability insurance in recent years, and would be unable to recoup any possible losses by insurance of subsequent programs because this is a one-time undertaking.

The initial proposal for the insurance pool was to provide $50 million worth of coverage for a possible $5 million straight premium for all four manufacturers. In the subsequent week the insurance industry worked with HEW and the manufacturers to try and actually develop the pool. They first found it necessary to steadily increase the price—first to a possible $25 million maximum retrospectively rated premium for $50 million of coverage and then to a possible $40 million maximum retrospectively rated premium which also included for the first time a potential profit of as much as $7 million in the event that losses did not exceed $33 million—and then proved unable at any of the prices to both obtain complete commitments to the pool and assurance of the availability of whatever necessary excess liability insurance would still be necessary.

Therefore, on August 2 HEW proposed a new approach to the problem because insurance was still not available, because it would clearly if available be extremely expensive, and because of increasing concern about liability problems for other participants in the program besides the vaccine manufacturers. This new approach, the tort claims approach, was considered by the Subcommittee on Health and the Environment in markups on August 3 and, after revision and polishing by the subcommittee, was ordered reported to the full Committee on Interstate and Foreign Commerce. The Committee on Interstate and Foreign Commerce met on August 5 to consider the legislation and directed that the chairman and staff of the Committee on the Judiciary be consulted with respect to it. This was done and their comments received on August 9 in the form of a letter to Chairman HARLEY O. STAGGERS from Chairman PETER RODINO of the Committee on the Judiciary, which I am attaching for the interest of the Members. This correspondence made several suggestions which have been adopted in the proposed legislation, indicated that the basic policy decisions were those of the Committee on Interstate and Foreign Commerce and said that the Committee on the Judiciary, in light of the emergency nature of the situation, would not seek sequential referral of the legislation. The Committee on Interstate and Foreign Commerce then met again today to consider the legislation further but adjourned due to the absence of a quorum.

THE TORT CLAIMS APPROACH

The "tort claims approach" recommended by HEW and adopted by the subcommittee is described in detail in the following section-by-section analysis. The legislation first provides authority for the program, requires reports from the Department on its implementation, and gives some direction to the Department with respect to the activities which should be included in it. With respect to liability arising out of the program, it then requires that people who assert claims arising out of injury or death attributable to inoculation with the vaccine in the program shall have as their exclusive remedy claim against the United States for that injury or death. These claims are to be made using the well-known, established procedures of the Federal Tort Claims Act, with certain exceptions described later, but are to be governed by the substance of the law of the place in which the claim accrues so that no one's rights are limited by the substitution of the United States as the party defendant. The United States is then given authority, in the event that it suffers loss on account of a claim because a participant in the program was negligent or failed to fulfill its contract obligations, to seek recovery of the losses from that program participant on this basis. This has the effect of leaving program participants at risk for damages caused by their negligence—or failure to produce a vaccine that meets contract specifications, which means that they will still need insurance against that possibility—but of protecting them against all meritless suits and generally against claims which arise out of concepts of liability that are not based on negligence. Preliminary indications have been received that, with the proposed legislation, the insurance industry will be able to provide the necessary insurance for program participants' residual liability, given that the meritless suits are handled by the Federal Government and that the liability is limited by the legislation.

This approach has been adopted because the Federal Government has initiated and fostered the swine flu program and assumed many of the responsibilities for the development of the vaccine and implementation of the program that might normally be handled in the private sector. Since the Government is also the purchaser of 100 percent of the output of the manufacturers, it has become the real party at interest for the program and it is therefore reasonable for it to assume, at least as a first principal, liability arising out of the program. Further, the approach has the advantage that it will not require additional appropriations, will almost certainly be less costly than allowing the insurance industry to handle the claims, uses an existing claims handling structure that includes authority on the part of the Government to settle small claims—less than $25,000—without delay, does not allow program participants to escape the responsibility for their own negligence or failures to discharge their obligations, and assures greater recoveries to injured claimants than likely under the private claims system because under the Federal Tort Claims Act attorneys' contingency fees are limited to a maximum of 20 percent of settled claims and 25 percent of recoveries after trial. The approach has the additional advantage that it will permit HEW to monitor swine flu adverse reactions directly without having to receive information on reactions indirectly from insurance carriers, other program participants, and vaccine recipients.

The tort claims approach does have possible drawbacks. In the unlikely event, in view of the known safety of the vaccine, that the possible large number of suits envisioned by the insurance industry does eventuate, it might be necessary to obtain authorization for additional staff for the handling of claims for HEW, and possibly the Justice Department. Further, the use of this approach relieves the insurance industry of many of its normal claims handling responsibilities in conjunction with programs such as this in the face of a clear feeling on the part of many Members that, were a way of holding the industry to the exercise of these responsibilities available, they should be so held.

The constitutionality of the remedial provisions of the legislation is firmly supported by judicial decisions which have upheld similar statutory schemes against constitutional challenges or merely applied such provisions without questioning their constitutionality. The Federal Drivers Act (18 U.S.C. 2679 (b)), for example, effectively abolished a pre-existing common law tort action against employees of the Federal Government for negligent driving by making an action against the Government under the Federal Tort Claims Act the exclusive remedy for persons injured by such activity. The Federal courts have upheld that statute against claims that its remedial scheme violated the due process clause of the fifth amendment and the seventh amendment right to trial by jury.[1] The courts have also routinely applied, without questioning their constitutionality, two similar statutes[2] which make a suit against the Government under the Tort Claims Act the exclusive remedy for persons injured by the alleged malpractice of physicians employed by the Veterans' Administration and the Public Health Service, respectively. Like those existing statutes, the present legislation substitutes a substantial and efficient remedy for the previous available common law remedy, in furtherance of a valid exercise of the legislative power.

The proposed legislation's constitutionality can also be seen in its similarity to 28 U.S.C. 1498 which provides that copyright and patent claims based upon activities of Government contractors may not be brought against those contractors and that instead the exclusive remedy is against the United States *(Richmond Screw Anchor Co. v. United States, 275 U.S. 331 (1928)),* and in the Supreme Court's recognition, in other contexts, that the Constitution does not forbid abolishing common law rights to attain permissible legislative objectives *(Silver v. Silver, 280 U.S.*

117 (1929); *New York Central RR Co.* v. *White,* 243 U.S. 188 (1916)).

The rationale for having a vaccine program in the first place requires that it be conducted no later than early fall and clearly continued debate and failure to resolve the liability problems is already beginning to delay the program into October. Delay of a decision until after the coming Congressional recess would certainly delay the program into November and expose the entire population to what must be considered a small but unacceptable risk of an epidemic. Thus it has been necessary to choose an approach to solving the liability problem which, while imperfect, will work, and to bring the debate to a close so that the program can proceed without further delay.

A section-by-section analysis and a letter follow:

SECTION-BY-SECTION ANALYSIS OF S.3735

The first section of S. 3735 provides that the Act may be cited as the "National Swine Flu Immunization Program of 1976." The second section amends section 317 of the Public Health Service Act (42 U.S.C. 247(b)) by adding after the existing last subsection, subsection (i), three new subsections. Section 317 of the PHS Act is the existing legislative authority, recently revised and extended by P.L. 94-317, for the prevention and control of disease by the Department of Health, Education, and Welfare. Historically, section 317 has been the principal Federal authority for the control of communicable diseases. It is also the principal current authority for immunization programs directed at the control of diphtheria, pertussis and tetanus (dpt), measles, polio, and rubella. These programs, all directed principally at children and conducted on an on-going basis, are essentially similar in their design to that of the proposed National Swine Flu Immunization Program. For these reasons the new authority for the swine flu program is located in existing section 317. It is the intent of the legislation that this authority become, effective upon its enactment, the sole authority for the conduct of the program. For this reason it has been designed to provide adequate authority for all facets of the program as they are presently understood. This should not be understood to mean that the vaccine and other materials to be used in the program are exempted from any other existing statutory requirements.

New paragraph (j)(1) authorizes the Secretary of Health, Education, and Welfare to establish, conduct, and support (by grant or contract) the activities needed to carry out a National Swine Flu Immunization Program.

The proposed legislation limits the authorized activities under the swine flu program to:

(A) The development of a safe and effective swine flu vaccine. Swine flu vaccine is defined by new paragraph (1) (3) as vaccine against the strain of influenza virus known as influenza A/New Jersey/76 (Hsw 1 Nsw 1) or a combination of such vaccine and the vaccine against the strain of influenza virus known as influenza A/Victoria/a/3/75 (H3N2). This is done because it is planned that the program will provide bivalent vaccine to the high-risk population so that the high-risk population will receive the protection against A/Victoria influenza virus which had already been planned prior to the identification of the swine flu variant. The high-risk population is understood to include individuals over 65, and people suffering from chronic lung disease, heart disease, diabetes, kidney disease, or other chronic diseases which affect pulmonary function.

(B) The preparation and procurement of the swine flu vaccine in sufficient quantities for the immunization of the population of the States. This subparagraph authorizes HEW to buy enough doses of swine flu vaccine for the entire United States population. It is not intended to commit the Secretary to buy that much vaccine. Certainly he should not purchase vaccine for any part of the population (such as young children) for which it proves impossible to establish a safe and effective dose. Further, after some experience with what fraction of the population actually seeks vaccination in the first States in which programs are undertaken, it should be possible to make some reduction in the number of doses purchased in anticipation of some percentage (hopefully small) of the U.S. population which chooses in a voluntary program such as this one not to be vaccinated. The government would remain obligated, however, to purchase all vaccine which it had actually committed itself by contract to purchase from the manufacturers. Since the program is designed to provide sufficient quantities of vaccine for all Americans who seek it, and since it can be anticipated that the States will make some vaccine available to private physicians and health programs to be used to vaccinate those who cannot receive vaccination in a public mass program, neither the monovalent swine flu vaccine nor the bivalent vaccine will be available in the normal private domestic market.

(C) The making of grants to State health authorities to assist in meeting their costs in conducting and supporting programs to administer the vaccine to their populations, and the furnishing to State health authorities of sufficient quantities of swine flu vaccine for their programs. This language does not require the Federal government to bear all of the costs of the State health authorities (and local agencies and organizations including local health departments to which the State authorities may subgrant or contract for assistance in the conduct of their programs). It is, however, the intent of the legislation that as large a fraction of these costs as possible be borne by the Federal government. However, the Committee recognizes that the $135 million appropriated to date may not be sufficient to cover the full costs of the program including those of the State and local health authorities. State and local costs in excess of the amounts provided in grants from the $135 million appropriation could be met out of State and local funds, from strictly voluntary contributions, or from additional Federal appropriations if necessary.

(D) The furnishing to Federal health authorities of appropriate quantities of such vaccine. The Federal government provides direct health care through the Department of Defense, Veterans Administration health care programs, and such smaller programs as the Indian Health Service. All of these should be provided sufficient quantities of the vaccine to protect the populations for whom they are responsible. The subcommittee noted with interest that the Veterans' Administration apparently lacks authority for a preventive health program such as the swine flu program since the authority for veterans' health care is for caring for existing diseases. The legislation does not include authority for such preventive health programs in the VA program because such authority would not be in the jurisdiction of the Committees of the House and Senate responsible for the proposed legislation and time was not available during consideration of the legislation for appropriate consideration by the Committee on Veterans Affairs. However, it is hoped that authority for at least the swine flu program can be found or provided to the veterans health care programs.

The military services—as is their custom—plan to use a more potent and more broadly constituted vaccine than will be used in the civilian program. Whereas most civilians will receive a small vaccine dose targeted solely against swine flu, the military services will administer a much larger dose with twice the the civilian dose targeted at swine flu and the remainder against two other flu strains. The primary purpose of the military immunization program is to conserve the nation's fighting force rather than to protect individuals, so the military puts greater emphasis on making certain that the vaccine is strong enough to provide protection. It is less concerned about possible side effects, unless those side effects threaten to disable the fighting force.

As one top military medical man put it, "Generally speaking, it's not at all intolerable for recruits to have a bad evening . . . They are febrile. They do feel lousy . . . A significant number of them are losing their meals as they come out of the mess. But they're back at work the next morning." (And they don't often file malpractice suits.) Because so much of the military population falls into the 18-to-24 age group that responded only to the "whole virus" type vaccines, the military will use only those in its program. One of the military's chosen vaccines caused temperatures of 100°F or more in 20 percent of the recipients and systemic reactions (headache, nausea, fever, and the like) in 31 percent.

(E) The conduct and support of training of personnel for the immunization activities described above and of research on the nature, cause and effect of the influenza against which the swine flu vaccine is designed to immunize, the nature and effects of the vaccine is designed to immunize, the nature and cine, immunization against and treatment of such influenza, and the cost and effects of immunization programs against such influenza. [sic.]

(F) The development, in consultation with the National Commission for the Protection of Human Subjects of Biomedical and Behavorial Research, and implementation of a written informed consent form and procedures for assuring that the risks and benefits from the swine flu vaccine are fully explained to each individual to whom such vaccine is to be administered. Such consultation is to be completed within two weeks after enactment of the legislation, or by September 1, 1976, whichever is sooner. The informed consent procedures are also to include information needed to advise individuals with respect to their rights and remedies arising out of any personal injuries or deaths resulting from the administration of the vaccine.

Since HEW is assuming full responsibility in this program for the duty to warn potential recipients of the vaccine of its possible risks and benefits, and to obtain from each recipient or his guardian his informed consent to such vaccination, and has, in the eyes of some, a bias in favor of its own program, it was felt necessary to require some independent scrutiny of the Department's proposed forms and procedures. Since the National Commission for the Protection of Human Subjects of Biomedical Research already exists and is aware of informed consent issues and procedures the legislation directs that it be consulted with respect to the forms and procedures proposed by the Department. It is understood that these must be completed and ready for use by sometime in September if their preparation is not to delay the program.

It is understood that each grant to the States to conduct the swine flu program includes a condition that they arrange to have the informed consent statement furnished to persons to whom vaccinations are to be administered. The informed consent form will advise such persons of the benefits of vaccinations and the possible side effects. It will contain special precautions for certain individuals, such as those allergic to eggs. It will advise any persons who believe they have claims for injury from inoculation with the vaccine that such claims must be filed against the United States, and on where to obtain information concerning the filing and handling of claims.

The requirement that recipients be informed of their rights and remedies in the event of injury is included because the legislation itself changes recipients' normal remedies in connection with this one specific program. There is no legislative intent to encourage litigation. To the contrary, the intent is to point out to individuals that this is a unique procedure and that their rights are established by this statute. Indeed, it is likely that suits under program will be diminished by including in the notice information regarding how to pursue administrative claims through the normal Federal tort claims procedures without initially having to undertake the legal costs normally required in situations where no administrative remedy is available.

(G) Such other activities as are necessary to implement the swine flu program. It is understood that it may be necessary for the Department to undertake activities which are not described in the previous paragraphs and have not yet been anticipated. Therefore this authority is given but it is anticipated that, if any activities not presently contemplated are undertaken, the Department will promptly inform the authorizing Committees with jurisdiction over the program with a detailed explanation of how and why new activities are being pursued.

New paragraph (j) (2) requires the Secretary of HEW to submit quarterly reports to the Congress on the administration of the swine flu program. It specifies that each such report is to provide information on:

(A) The current supply of the swine flu vaccine to be used in the program.

(B) The number of people inoculated with the vaccine since the last report was made and the immune status of the population. Reports on the immune status of the population should make clear what parts of the population are protected to what extend against exposure to the swine flu virus. Doing this will require specification of standards and measures of immunity and some sampling of the population to establish antibody titer levels from both inoculation with the vaccine and prior infection with the swine flu virus. Reports of the immune status of the population should consider such factors as the rates at which different parts of the population are obtaining inoculation, the herd effect, the time required to develop immunity after inoculation, and the population's response to the vaccine.

(C) The amount of funds expended for the swine flu program by the United States, each State, and any other entity participating in the program and the costs of each such participant which are associated with the program, during the period with respect to which the report is made. This requirement is intended to require HEW to undertake formal public costs that drug manufacturers experience in producing the vaccine, including the costs of insurance which they purchase or otherwise incur for their participation in the program, the amounts of public expenditures experienced by State and local entities from sources other than grants made under the program, and litigation costs experienced by HEW and the Department of Justice in connection with the administration of new section 317 (k), described below.

(D) The epidemiology of influenza in the United States during the period covered by the report. This aspect of the report should describe the epidemiology of all strains of influenza identifiable in the United States, not only the swine flu strain. It should describe the incidence of the disease as well as its effects on those infected and its movement in the United States population.

These quarterly reports should begin immediately upon enactment, with the first report covering the history of the program in each of the areas specified since the decision to initiate the program was made by the President in March of this year. Reports should continue as long as funds obligated from the appropriation made by P. L. 49-266 have not been outlayed, or contractual obligations under contracts written in connection with the program are outstanding. If reporting by these criteria becomes necessary for more than a year it would be appropriate for reports at yearly intervals to summarize the preceding year.

It would also be appropriate for the Department to combine the reporting requirements of this new subparagraph (j) (2) with those of new section 317 (k) (8). This would avoid the additional cost in making two separate reports but would require coordination of the reporting activity between the Department of HEW and the Department of Justice since the latter is likely to share responsibility for the reporting requirement in section 317 (k) (8).

New paragraph 317 (j) (3) requires any contract by the Federal government or procurement by it of swine flu vaccine from any vaccine manufacturer to (notwithstanding any other provision of law) be subject to renegotiation to eliminate any profit realized from the procurement. Profit and the methods to be used for renegotiation are to be determined pursuant to criteria prescribed by the Secretary. An exception is provided which would allow profit to be made on vaccine against A/Victoria 75 influenza but limit that profit to no more than reasonable profit. Provisions for renegotiation are to be expressly included in the contracts and they (and the Secretary's criteria) are to specify that any insurance premium included in the costs for the manufacturer of the vaccine which is refunded to the manufacturer under a retrospective, experience rating insurance plan or a similar such rating plan shall in turn be refunded to the United States.

In view of the unusual insulation being provided the drug manufacturers against costs of defending suits to which they would normally be a party, and since express indications had been given of willingness to provide the vaccine on a nonprofit basis by representatives of all four of the manufacturers, the legislation includes the requirement that profit be eliminated from the sale of the swine flu vaccine. This should of course be facilitated and demonstrated by the cost accounting required by new subparagraph 317 (j) (2) (C).

Profit is permitted with respect to the A-Victoria 75 vaccine because it was made before the program was initiated in anticipation of profit by the manufacturers who will not, by the design of the program, be permitted to market it in the normal fashion. Thus it seems reasonable to permit the anticipated profit with respect to the one vaccine while precluding it with respect to the other.

It is hoped that insurance for this program can also be purchased on a nonprofit basis, perhaps through a retrospective rating form of insurance or some other form in which the premium is adjusted after the fact to reflect actual experience under the policy. Whether or not a retrospective plan permitted a profit to the insurors, to the extent that such a plan is used the premiums refunded to the drug manufacturer would also be refunded by them to the United States.

Direct reference to the publication of regulations for this provision is avoided so that the long delays normally encountered by the Department in preparation of regulations will not delay the program. It is understood that the criteria to be used by the Secretary in determining costs and "reasonable" profits will be made known to the manufacturers before they must submit their formal contract bids.

New paragraph 317 (j) (4) specifies that appropriations are not authorized for the program (and thus are also not available from any other authority) in addition to those already appropriated by P. L. 94-266, a total of $135 million. Exceptions to this general rule are made for State grants and unanticipated activities (subparagraphs (C) and (G) of 317 (j) (1), respectively) as described above.

The limitation on authorizations for appropriations is designed to assure that further public funds are not used for the program without the need for them being established before the authorizing Committees and approved by those Committees.

New paragraph 317 (k) (1) contains Congressional findings in subparagraph 317 (k) (1) (A) and a statement of Congressional purpose in subparagraph 317 (k) (1) (B) respecting the procedure established by new section 317 (k) for the handling of claims for personal injury or death arising out of the administration of the swine flu vaccine.

Specifically, the Congress finds that:

(i) In order to achieve the participation in the program of the agencies, organizations and individuals who will manufacture, distribute and administer the swine flu vaccine purchased and used in the program, and to assure the availability of the vaccine in interstate commerce, it is necessary to protect the agencies, organizations and individuals against liability to persons alleging personal injury or death arising out of the administration of the vaccine except for liability arising out of any negligence on the part of the agencies, organizations and individuals involved.

(ii) To provide such protection against liability and to establish an orderly procedure for the prompt handling of claims by persons alleging injury or death arising from the administration of vaccine, it is necessary that an exclusive remedy for such claimants be provided against the United States because of its unique role in the initiation, planning and administration of the swine flu program.

(iii) In order to be prepared to meet the potential emergency of a swine flu epidemic (which, were it similar to the epidemic in 1918-19, would genuinely constitute a national emergency, since it would close schools and work places and swamp the nation's health system while reducing the strength of its defenses), it is necessary that a procedure be instituted for the handling of claims by persons alleging injury or death in connection with the program until Congress can develop a more permanent approach for handling claims which arise out of other public medical programs conducted under the authority of the Public Health Service Act, to the extent that any permanent solution to any of the problems proves necessary.

These findings are based on the refusal of the insurance industry to include the swine flu vaccine under the four manufacturers' normal product liability insurance, because of their belief that the unusual size of the program and publicity connected with it would result in a multiplicity of suits against multiple defendants which, whether meritless or ultimately successful against any of the defendants, would be costly to defend. It was believed that defendants would undergo substantial costs just to protect their interests in these suits. A similar situation threatened to develop with insurers of health care providers who might participate in administering the vaccine.

The findings are made only after a two-month effort by the House Subcommittee on Health and the Environment and HEW to find some other approach to the handling of liability, either without legislation or with legislation using a different approach. These efforts included the specification in the contract with the manufacturers that the government was assuming, for this one program, obligations, such as the duty to warn and the development of vaccine specifications, which are normally carried out by the manufacturer in other immunization programs. However, these efforts offered no other conclusion but that this legislation was necessary if the program proposed by the President was to be carried forward with the cooperation of the vaccine manufacturers and the insurance industry in an expeditious manner.

It is found necessary to provide an exclusive remedy against the United States in order to "channel" all liability under the program into one forum, against one defendant, and so avoid the insurers' defense costs entailed in weeding out who is the proper defendant and a multiplicity of meritless claims. The use of the Federal Tort Claims Act to provide an exclusive remedy for claimants under certain circumstances is not unique. Several other statutes provide partial or complete immunity to certain Federal employees by invoking the procedures of the Federal Tort Claims Act. See 28 U.S.C. 2679 (b)-(e): 38 U.S.C. 4116; 42 U.S.C. 233 (c); P. L. 94–350. The Department of Justice has assured the Chairman of the Judiciary Committee that from their point of view "there is an abundance of legislative and court decision precedent" and that "the statutes upon which the bill is patterned have provided a very efficient and effective means for disposing of claims."

By using its existing procedures for processing tort claims, HEW could dispose of a number of such claims administratively with relatively little delay.

These findings demonstrate that the remedial provisions of the legislation are necessary and proper measures in furtherance of Congressional power to regulate with respect to a vaccine which is to be distributed in interstate commerce and to protect the public welfare against a possible national emergency. The findings also make it clear that the approach chosen is limited entirely to the specific swine flu immunization program authorized by the legislation. Further, the findings convey the understanding that the approach chosen might not have been considered the most meritorious in other situations and is not intended to prejudice debate over the possible need for legislation (and the approach to be taken by that legislation) in other circumstances. It is hoped that once the insurance industry and program participants have the experience of such a nationwide program, the experience and data gathered can be used as a guide to prevent similar problems from occurring in other such immunization programs.

Subparagraph 317 (k) (1) (B) states that it is the purpose of subsection 317 (k) to establish the procedure found necessary as described in subparagraph 317 (k) (1) (A) under which all claims are to be asserted directly against the United States under section 1346 (b) of title 28 U.S.C. in chapter 171 of such title (the Federal Tort Claims Act) except as is otherwise specifically provided in subsection 317 (k). This purpose is pursued in order to:

i. assure an orderly procedure for the prompt, equitable handling of any claim for personal injury or death arising out of the administration of the vaccine;

ii. to achieve the participation in the program of the manufacturers and distributors of the vaccine, public and private agencies or organizations providing the vaccine without charge and in compliance with informed consent forms and procedures, and medical and other health professionals providing the vaccine or assisting in doing so without charge and in compliance with the required consent forms and procedures.

The procedures of the Federal Tort Claims Act are chosen because they are well known and established. As described below, the liability of the United States will be governed by the law of the State where the act or omission causing injury occurred.

New paragraph 317 (k) (2) makes the United States liable with respect to claims submitted after September 30, 1976, for personal injury or death arising out of the administration of swine flu vaccine under the swine flu program which are based upon the act or omission of a program participant. The liability arises only after September 30, in order to avoid conflict with the Congressional Budget Act. This is not expected to cause difficulty or delay because it is understood that the program has already been delayed by the debate over the legislation to the point that it is unlikely that inoculations will be given before the beginning of October.

The protection of section 317 (k) extends to all "program participants," a term that is defined in subparagraph 317 (k) (2) (B) to include manufacturers and distributors of the vaccine, as well as public and private agencies and medical and other health personnel who both provide an inoculation without charge to the recipient and who comply with the applicable requirements for obtaining informed consent. The phrase "without charge for the vaccine or its administration" in subsection 317 (k) (2) (B) is intended to exclude from the coverage of the Act agencies or medical personnel who charge the recipient for an inoculation. The phrase is not intended to deny protection under the legislation to the regular and temporary medical and para-medical employees of public or private organizations who receive their regular salaries and wages while participating in the program and who do not charge the public for their services. It is not intended that State and local health departments would be precluded from collecting voluntary contributions for the provision of the vaccine as long as they are explicitly and clearly voluntary.

A private agency or organization as intended in the definition would include any hospital, school system, church, or other health care institution or social agency, employer, or other organization which provided an inoculation. Program participants are defined on a claim-by-claim basis so that the failure of a program participant such as a State to give an individual injection of the vaccine either without charge or in compliance with the informed consent forms and procedures requirements would not prevent such a participant from being covered by the protection of the legislation as a program participant in connection with a claim arising from another inoculation which was given both without charge and in compliance with the informed consent requirements.

It should be noted that one of the problems that the government may have under the program will be knowing which of the drug manufacturers to claim against if they wish to make such a claim. In this connection, it is hoped that the Department will make every effort in implementing the program to provide record keeping systems which allow identification of the lot from which the vaccine provided to each individual inoculated was taken.

The intent of subparagraph 317 (k) (2) is that the substantive tort law of the jurisdiction where the act or omission occurred shall govern any action brought against the United States for injuries based on the act or omission of a program participant. However, the Federal Tort Claims Act limits the right to sue the United States, primarily by limiting suits to those based on negligence, and by exempting from liability discretionary actions taken by United States officials. Therefore, several exceptions are specified to the rule that the United States is to be liable with respect to claims based upon the act or omission of a program participant in the same manner and extent as it would be in other actions brought against it under the Federal Tort Claims Act. These exceptions specify that:

I. The liability of the United States arising out of the act or omission of a program participant may be based on any theory of liability that would govern an action against such program participant under the law of the place where the act or omission occurred, including negligence, strict liability in tort, and breach of warranty.

The effect, of this provision is that the terms of 28 U.S.C. 1346 (b) for purposes of the swine flu program are modified so that liability of the United States is not determined "under circumstances where the United States, if a private person, would be liable," but rather under circumstances where a program participant would be liable under State law at the time the case arose.

The purpose of (k) (2) (A) (i) was to make explicit that the United States would defend each action as though it were taking place in a State court where the claim arose and governed by the law of that State. Thus, to the extent that a program participant would have been subject to suit under the law of the State where the act or omission occurred, the United States will be similarly subject to suit, without respect to the legal theory upon which the suit is based. Similarly, the United States, which stands in the shoes of the program participant for the purposes of suit, should plead any defenses which then exist under State law including the terms of the tort claims acts of the individual States and of any statute and common law immunizing program participants from liability from suit.

In short, the Act creates no new cause of action in favor of claimants, but merely establishes a new procedure for vindicating such claims as the claimants could have made under the terms of their own State law against State governmental entities or program participants.

It should be noted here that section 317 (k) (7) of the Act, discussed below, is designed to govern the United States' right to indemnification from program participants only after the liability of the United States has been established under State law. The phrase "notwithstanding any provision of State law" in that paragraph was simply intended only to assure that certain State joint tortfeasor contribution laws would not prevent the United States' claim over against a program participant.

II. The discretionary function exemption specified in section 2680 (a) of title 28 U.S.C. will not be available to the United States in defending claims against it based upon the act or omission of a program participant. Note here that the United States is not a program participant as defined in subsection 317 (k) (2) (B) and thus that actions against it based on acts or omission of the United States will be governed by the normal terms and procedures of the Federal Tort Claims Act. Thus the discretionary function exemption would be available to the United States against claims made directly against it but not with respect to claims made against the United States in lieu of other program participants. This was again done out of a desire to neither limit nor broaden the substantive rights of plaintiffs under existing law.

iii. If a civil action or proceeding for personal injury or death arising out of the administration of the vaccine under the program is brought within two years of the date of the administration of the vaccine and is dismissed because the plaintiff in the action did not file an administrative claim with respect to the injury or death as required by chapter 171, the plaintiff in the action or proceeding is to have at least 30 days from the date of such dismissal (or two years from the date the claim arose, whichever is later) in which to file the required administrative claim (notwithstanding the provisions of section 2041 (b) of title 28 U.S.C. which otherwise limits the time for the filing of claims to two years). This provision, recommended by the Chairman of the House Committee on the Judiciary, is intended to assure that no claimant under the program would be barred by the statute of limitations from filing a tort claim against the United States simply because he or she filed a suit against a program participant in State court instead of utilizing the Federal Tort Claims Act procedures.

New paragraph 317 (k) (3) specifies that the remedy against the

United States prescribed by new paragraph 317 (k) (2) (and described above) for personal injury or death arising out of the administration of the vaccine under the program is to be exclusive of any other civil action or proceeding for such injury or death against any employee of the government (as defined in section 2671 of title 28 U.S.C.) or program participant whose act or omission gave rise to the claim for which the remedy is available.

The remedies of paragraph 317 (k) (2) are made exclusive principally because the manufacturers and insurors would not agree to participate unless the manufacturers were insulated from the spurious lawsuits they expected to ensue. For these same reasons authority is not provided for the Federal government to implead program participants as third party defendants in suits which would otherwise be brought against the program participants. Were the program participants impleaded they would then bear the cost of defending themselves and would need insurance against those costs. All of this, of course, arises from the perceived risk on the part of the drug manufacturers, their insurers, and other program participants that there will be numerous suits filed in connection with the program which (even if they prove nonmeritorious or properly directed against another defendant) will impose costly litigation burdens upon the program participants which might prove uninsurable.

New paragraph 317 (k) (4) requires the Attorney General to defend any civil action or proceeding brought in any court against any employee of the government (as defined in section 2671) or program participant (or any liability insurer of a program participant in a State in which claims may be made against an insurer directly as well as against those whom the insurer insures, such as Florida and Louisiana) based upon a claim alleging personal injury or death arising out of the administration of the vaccine under the program. Any person against whom civil actions or proceedings are brought is to deliver all process served upon him (or an attested true copy thereof) to whoever is designated by the Secretary to receive the papers and process, and any such person is to promptly furnish copies of the pleadings and process therein to the United States attorney for the district embracing the place where the civil action or proceeding is brought, to the Attorney General and to the Secretary of HEW.

New paragraph 317 (k) (5) (A) specifies that a civil action or proceeding brought in any court against any employee of the government or a program participant which is based upon a claim alleging personal injury or death is to be deemed an action against the United States under the provisions of title 28 U.S.C. (and all references thereto) upon certification by the Attorney General that the civil action or proceeding is in fact based upon such a claim. If the action is originally brought in a district court of the United States, then upon certification by the Attorney General as provided above the United States is further to be substituted as the party defendant in the action or proceeding.

New subparagraph 317 (k) (5) (b) provides that upon the same certification by the Attorney General described above with respect to a civil action or proceeding commenced in a State court, the action or proceeding is to be removed, without bond and at any time before trial, by the Attorney General to the appropriate district court of the United States. The appropriate district court is that of the district in the division embracing the place wherein the civil action or proceeding is pending. Actions or proceedings thus removed will also thereby be deemed an action or proceeding brought against the United States under the provisions of title 28 U.S.C. (and all references thereto) and the United States will be substituted as the party defendant in the action or proceeding.

The Attorney General's certification with respect to an individual's or organization's program participant status is to conclusively establish such status for the purpose of initial removal to the Federal district court and substitution of the United States as party defendant. If the district court determines, after such removal and substitution, on a hearing on a motion to remand held before the trial on the merits, that an action or proceeding is not one to which the subsection applies, the case is to be remanded to the State court.

The determination that subsection 317 (k) does not apply to a particular claim would usually be made on the grounds that in the particular case in question the vaccine was given with charge or the would-be program participant administering the vaccine had failed to fulfill his obligation to obtain informed consent. In such cases once this finding of fact was made by the district court the individual or organization would lose its status as a program participant and be substituted back as defendant in the action or proceeding, which would then be remanded to the appropriate court. It is understood that claims may allege that charges were made or proper informed consent not obtained when they are first brought into State court and that it may be argued that this means that the defendant is not a program participant and the case should not be removed to Federal court. The intent of the legislation is that where a question of charge or informed consent is at issue in a claim, the claim shall be removed to Federal court for resolution of the issue. This is again intended to protect the defendants against bearing the cost of defense except in the event that their failure to comply with the requirement of section 317 (k) is established.

New subparagraph 317 (k) (5) (C) specifies that where an action or proceeding under this subsection is precluded because of availability of a remedy through proceedings for compensation or other benefits from the United States as provided by any other law, the action or proceeding shall be dismissed. However, in the event that such an action or proceeding is dismissed, the running of any time limitation for commencing or filing an application or claim in such proceedings for compensation or benefits is to be deemed to have been suspended during the pendency of the civil action or proceeding originally initiated under subsection 317 (k). This provision gives priority to the handling of claims, for which a remedy from the United States (as compared to some other source) is already available, using that remedy rather than the remedy provided by the legislation.

New subparagraph 317 (k) (6) requires program participants to cooperate with the United States in the processing and defense of a claim or suit under section 1346 (b) and chapter 171 based upon the alleged acts or omissions of the program participants. Upon the motion of the United States or of any other party to the civil action or proceeding arising out of the claim, the status as a program participant is to be revoked by the district court of the United States upon a finding by it that the program participant has failed to cooperate as required. In the event that program participant status is revoked, the court is to substitute the former participant as the party defendant in the place of the United States and, upon motion, remand any such suit, civil action or proceeding to the court in which it was originally instituted.

These provisions are designed to assure full cooperation of any program participants in the United States' defense of them under the provisions of the legislation and to provide a sanction which will assure this cooperation, to wit the possible loss of program participant status and thus the need for the program participant to defend itself in the claim or proceeding. The required cooperation is to extend to all normal discovery procedures available against the United States as the defendant in the action, subject of course to any privilege which can be asserted by the United States or derivatively on the part of a program participant. For example, interrogatories and requests for admissions of facts and genuineness of documents on the part of a program participant pursuant to the Federal Rules of Civil Procedure would be submitted to the United States for immediate delivery to the program participant. If the interrogatories or requests for admissions went unanswered within the 30-day limit of the Rules, the program participant, having failed to cooperate, would be subject to loss of its status as such. The required cooperation shall also extend to reasonable requirements made of program participants for information and documents necessary for adjudication of administrative claims. Notwithstanding the legislation's requirement for cooperation in discovery directed against the United States, a program participant would be subject to discovery by any party to the action regarding matter relevant to the subject matter of the action, as provided under the Federal Rules of Civil Procedure. The subpoena power of Rule 45 and the sanctions of Rule 37 are available for the purposes of such discovery.

New subparagraph 317 (k) (7), creates a Federal cause of action by the United States against a program participant in which the United States could recover any amount it had paid by settlement or judgment as well as costs of litigation and settlement "resulting from the failure of any program participant to carry out any obligation or responsibility assumed by it under a contract with the United States in connection with the program or from any negligent conduct on the part of any program participant in carrying out any obligation or responsibility in connection with the swine flu program." The cause of action is conditioned upon the United States making payment, and thus the cause of action accrues upon the making of such payment. The United States is given authority to maintain actions against program participants for recovery of damages in the district court of the United States in which the program participant resides or has its principal place of business.

The phrase "notwithstanding any provision of state law" has been included on the recommendation of the Chairman of the Committee on the Judiciary, and is intended to make clear that the United States' right of recovery over against program participants shall not be precluded by laws, existing in many States, barring suits for contribution among joint tortfeasors. In this way, the fact that a suit had initially been brought, for example, based both on a claim that a lot of vaccine was both defectively manufactured and negligently inspected by the government would not prevent the government from later seeking recovery for any damages it paid based on defective manufacture. The phrase is not intended to affect the substantive State law of liability for the acts or omissions of program participants, including any State law of immunity from suit for any such program participants. As discussed above with reference to paragraph 317 (k) (2), the intent of the legislation is to leave State law in this regard unchanged, with the United States standing in the shoes of the program participant for the purposes of suit, and thus derivatively entitled to immunity.

The right of the United States is "to recover for that portion of the damages so awarded or paid, as well as any costs of litigation." Because the language refers to the "portion" of the amount paid which is the result of the participant's acts or omissions, it is the clear intention that the participant could not contend that the United States was barred from recovery because of any alleged negligence by the United States. Rather, the United States could recover for whatever portion of the amount paid could be shown to have resulted from the program participant's failure to carry out its obligations and responsibilities under the program. This type of proportional recovery is similar to that recognized by the Supreme Court in *United States* v. *Seckinger,* 397 U.S. 203 (1970).

It is generally anticipated that the United States will use this right of recovery in any situation in which damages for which it has been held liable were caused by the negligence of a program participant or by a program participant's failure to carry out one of its obligations or responsibilities. The authority is discretionary because it is recognized that there may be occasional situations in which the amount of damages which could be recovered is not worth the cost or in which the United States clearly cannot hope to establish the program participant's negligence or responsibility. However, it is expected that these will be unusual situations on which the Secretary will report to the Congress with an explanation of why the authority has not been used.

The bases for liability for recovery over by the United States are two: "the failure of any program participant to carry out any obligation or responsibility assumed by it under a contract with the United States in connection with the program," and "any negligent conduct on the part of any program participant in carrying out any obligation or responsibility in connection with the swine flu program."

With regard to the first of these, if production of the product was not in accordance with the specifications furnished by the government, or if it was contaminated, the United States would not have to show the specific negligence that resulted in the contamination. Rather, the United States need only prove that the original plaintiff's damages were caused by the program participant's failure to comply with the government's specifications or other contractual obligations assumed by it under a contract entered into in connection with the program.

With regard to the second basis for liability, the provision is not intended to give the United States the right to recover against others for failure by the United States to perform its own obligations and responsibilities in connection with the program. Thus, for example, since the United States is assuming from the drug manufacturers the duty to warn, in the case of damages arising out of failure to warn a recipient of the vaccine of its possible risks the United States would not be able to recover from the drug manufacturers for damages paid on that basis. With respect to manufacturers of the vaccine, the phrase "any obligation or responsibility in connection with the program" includes all actions in connection with the manufacture and distribution of the vaccine other than actions involving a duty specifically assumed by the United States under the program.

New subparagraph 317 (k) (8) requires a report within a year after the enactment of the legislation, and semi-annually thereafter, from the Secretary to the Congress on the conduct of settlement and litigation activities under subsection 317 (k). The report is to specify the number, value, nature and status of all claims made under the subsection and to include a description of the status of claims for recovery by the United States against program participants for damages made under paragraph 317 (k) (7) (with detailed explanation of the reasons for not seeking such recovery in any situation in which it is not sought).

New section 317 (1) defines certain terms for the purposes of new subsection 317 (j) and (k). Specifically, the phrase "arising out of the administration" with reference to a claim for personal injury or death under the swine flu program is to include a claim with respect to the manufacture or distribution of the vaccine in connection with the provision of an inoculation using it in swine flu program; the term "state" is to include the District of Columbia, Puerto Rico, the Virgin Islands, Guam, American Samoa and the Trust Territory of the Pacific Islands; and the term "swine flu vaccine" is to mean the vaccine against the strain of influenza virus known as influenza A/New Jersey/76 (Hsw 1N1), or a combination of that vaccine against the strain of influenza virus known as influenza A/Victoria/75.

Section 3 of the legislation directs the Secretary of HEW to conduct, or provide for the conduct of, a study of the scope and extent of liabilities for personal injuries or death arising out of immunization programs generally, and of alternative approaches to providing protection against such liability and/or compensation for such injuries. The report is due within a year after the enactment of the legislation and is to include the findings of the study, and whatever recommendations for legislation the Secretary deems appropriate.

It is the intention of the legislation that the report consider at least several major alternative approaches to the problem of injury and death arising out of public immunization programs. These would include public indemnification of private parties (as proposed by HEW in its original legislation in connection with the swine flu program), public reinsurance of private insurors of liability arising out of immunization programs, tort claims approaches such as that used by the legislation, and direct systems of compensation of injured parties for their injury without respect to the fault for the injury. The report to the Congress is intended to include actual draft legislation for the implementation by the Federal government of each of these alternative approaches to the problem with commentary on the merits and deficiencies of each approach and an indication of which is preferable in the judgment of the Secretary (if in his judgment any is necessary). If the report recommends adoption of an alternative to the current system, it should identify in detail, with supporting data, the inadequacies of the current system. It would be reasonable for the report to consider related reliability issues such as the liability that arises out of injuries or death experienced by voluntary participants in publicly funded medical research programs, and the liability that arises out of allergic reactions to drugs and biologicals absent any negligence on the part of the manufacturer, distributor or provider of the drug or biological in question.

CONGRESS OF THE UNITED STATES, COMMITTEE ON THE JUDICIARY,
Washington, D.C., August 9, 1976.

HON HARLEY O. STAGGERS, *Chairmen, Interstate and Foreign Commerce Committee, Rayburn House Office Building, Washington, D.C.*

Dear MR. CHAIRMAN: I am writing in response to your request for comment on H.R. 15050, the swine flu inoculation program bill. There has been no formal consideration of the bill by the Committee on the Judiciary, since the bill has not been referred to the Committee and there is thus nothing before it. However, I am pleased to advise you that I have consulted with numerous Members of the Judiciary Committee, including Congressman Walter Flowers, Chairman of the Subcommittee on Administrative Law and Governmental Relations, to which the bill would be referred if it came to the Judiciary Committee, and Congressman Ed Hutchinson, the ranking minority Member of the full Committee, and that my comments reflect their input. In addition, I have met with and sought the formal positions of the Departments of Justice and Health, Education and Welfare and have asked the staff of the Judiciary Committee, including those especially knowledgeable with respect to the Federal Tort Claims Act, to analyze the bill from a technical and legal point of view.

It is my understanding that you are principally interested in our opinion upon the manner in which the bill invokes the procedures of the Tort Claims Act to provide a means of processing claims for death or personal injury arising from the inoculation of citizens with the swine flu vaccine and of defining the liability to persons suffering such death or injury. The bill would provide that all such claims would be brought in the first instance against the United States government, which would establish an administrative claims procedure under the auspices of the Department of Health, Education and Welfare. If no administrative settlement is reached, suit against the government would be authorized under the normal procedures of the Tort Claims Act. Suits brought initially in state court against program participants would be removed to federal court by the Attorney General, with the United States substituted as the party defendant. Likewise, the United States would be substituted as the party defendant in all suits brought directly in federal court against program participants. Recovery against the government could be had under any tort theory, including strict liability or breach of warranty, available under the law of the state where the act or omission complained of occurred. In any case where it paid a settlement or judgment to a claimant, the federal government would then have a right of recovery over against any program participant for that amount of the damages attributable to the participant's acts or omissions of a negligent nature.

The net upshot of the bill is that the federal government would absorb the cost of processing and defending all unsuccessful claims and of satisfying all claims based on any theory of liability which did not involve negligence. To achieve this objective the bill would invoke the Tort Claims Act in an unusual, though not unique, manner. I am informed by Secretary Matthews of HEW that without the protection afforded program participants against the risks of litigation and its attendant costs by the bill, there would likely be no adequate government-sponsored swine flu inoculation program, since there would be no adequate insurance available. The policy judgment whether to afford this much protection at federal expense to those participating in the program in order to ensure that there is in fact an effective inoculation effort is in the first instance within the purview of the Committee on Interstate and Foreign Commerce, and I shall confine my comments to the legal aspects of the vehicle through which the bill seeks to achieve this objective.

As I noted above, the bill invokes the Tort Claims Act in an unusual, though not unique, manner. The bill makes no changes in the Tort Claims Act, and has no impact on it, except that in the narrow circumstances of suits under the bill, the government would waive the discretionary act exemption of the Tort Claims Act and would open itself to liability in the absence of negligence. Both provisions seem appropriate in the circumstances.

Several other statutes have invoked the procedures of the Tort Claims Act in a similar fashion to provide partial or complete immunity to certain kinds of federal employees. See 28 U.S.C. § 2679 (b)–(e); 38 U.S.C. § 4116; 42 U.S.C. § 233 (c); P.L. 94–350. Thus the Department of Justice assures me that from their point of view "there is an abundance of legislative and court decision precedent" and that "the statutes upon which the bill is patterned have provided a very efficient and effective means for disposing of claims." Nonetheless, I would be disturbed to see this mechanism invoked as a commonplace to relieve private individuals, companies and other non-federal entities of their normal responsibilities in situations where the federal government has an interest in promoting their participation. I believe, however, that the bill as drafted and its legislative history reflect appropriate emphasis upon the uniqueness of the government's role in promoting the swine flu vaccination program as the major, if not the sole, justification for this extraordinary procedure.

I do have some technical concern which could be accommodated with minor amendments. First, when a case is removed from state court to federal court under the bill and the United States is substituted as the party defendant, the case would be subject to a motion to dismiss if the plaintiff had failed to exhaust the administrative claims procedure to be established by HEW. This would cause no problem where there was ample time to run on the statutory limitation period of two years for the filing of the administrative claim. If, however, that period had expired prior to the removal and dismissal of the suit, the plaintiff could be left without a remedy, even though he had filed his suit in state court in timely fashion. I would suggest that in the event of such a removal and dismissal, the bill should provide the plaintiff with a minimum of thirty days in which to file his administrative claim. This could be accomplished by inserting the following language at the end of subsection 5 (b), dealing with removal of state court actions:

"Notwithstanding section 2401 (b) of title 28, United States Code, if a civil action or proceeding for personal injury or death resulting from the administration of vaccine under the Program is brought within two years of the date of the administration of the vaccine and is dismissed because the plaintiff in such action or proceeding did not file an administrative claim with respect to such injury or death as required by such chapter 171, the plaintiff in such action or proceeding shall have 30 days from the date of such dismissal or two years from the date the claim accrued, whichever is later, in which to file such administrative claim."

Second, there is a somewhat disturbing ambiguity in subsection (7) of the bill, which provides for the government's right of recovery over against program participants for their negligent acts or omissions contributing to the injury for which a payment has been made. The substantive law governing the original claimant's right of recovery is explicitly state law. The law of many states bars suits for contribution among joint tortfeasors. It is easy to conceive of cases in which the government would defend the initial suit both in its capacity as surrogate defendant for program participants and in the role of one of the alleged tortfeasors—for example, where a claim is made that a batch of vaccine was negligently manufactured by a drug company and negligently inspected by the government. The bill seems to me to leave room in that instance for the program participant to argue that state law would bar any recovery over by the government under subsection (7). I would suggest that an appropriate amendment be made to clarify the intent of the legislation and to provide that state law barring contribution among joint tortfeasors would not bar recovery by the government against a negligent program participant in such circumstances. This could be accomplished by wording subsection (7) to read as follows:

"(7) Should payment be made by the United States to any claimant bringing a claim under this subsection, either by way of administrative settlement or court judgment, the United States shall have, notwithstanding any provision of State law, a right of action to recover that portion of the damages so awarded or paid, as well as any costs of litigation, resulting from any negligent act or omission on the part of any Program participant in carrying out any obligation or responsibility in connection with the Program. The United States may maintain such action against such Program participant in the district court of the

United States in which such Program participant resides or has its principal place of business."

In conclusion, let me emphasize that the views expressed herein are my own, and not those of the Judiciary Committee expressed in any institutional manner. Let me further reiterate that I believe the fundamental policy choice at the core of this bill is one to be made in the first instance by the Committee on Interstate and Foreign Commerce, and I express no views on that issue. Having said that, it is my intention not to seek a sequential referral of this bill on behalf of the Judiciary Committee. The measure has the support of the White House, the Department of Justice and HEW, and both the President and the Secretary of HEW have urged that the matter be considered with all possible speed in view of the lead time necessary for the production and distribution of the vaccine. In view of these time problems and of your greatly appreciated courtesy in affording me this opportunity to express our legal opinion and technical concerns, I do not believe the public interest would be served by a sequential referral.

I hope these views are of some assistance to you, and I assure you that we stand ready to assist in whatever way we can, should you have any further questions.

With all best wishes,
    Sincerely,

PETER W. RODINO, JR.,
        Chairman.

[1] E.g., *Carr* v. *United States*, 422 F. 2d 1007 (4th Cir. 1970); *Nistendirk* v. *McGee*, 225 F. Supp. 881 (W.D. Mo. 1963).

[2] 38 U.S.C. § 4116, analyzed and applied in *Henderson* v. *Bluemink*, 511 F. 2d 399 (D.C. Cir. 1974) and *Smith* v. *DiCara*, 329 F. Supp. 438 (E.D.N.Y. 1971); and 42 U.S.C. § 233, applied in *Byrd* v. *Warden Federal Detention Headquarters*, 376 F. Supp. 37 (S.D.N.Y. 1974).

The Contributors

JUNE E. OSBORN, M.D., is a virologist and pediatrician who began doing virology research during her medical school years at (Case) Western Reserve University, where she received her M.D. in 1961. Subsequently she did three years of pediatric residency at Massachusetts General Hospital and Children's Hospital Medical Center in Boston, and then did two years of further postdoctoral training in infectious disease and virology at Johns Hopkins and the University of Pittsburgh. She is currently Professor of Medical Microbiology and Pediatrics at the University of Wisconsin Medical School in Madison, Wisconsin, where she has been on the faculty since 1966. Since 1975 she has also been Associate Dean for Biological Sciences of the University of Wisconsin Graduate School at Madison.

Dr. Osborn has done virology research and taught microbiology and infectious disease to medical students throughout her professional career. Since 1973 she has served as one of a seven-member Panel on Viral and Rickettsial Vaccines which is advisory to the Bureau of Biologics of the U.S. Food and Drug Administration. It was in this role, in 1976, that she became involved in the discussions leading to the "swine flu" program as one of the government's advisors. Since that time she has also served as a member of the Assistant Secretary for Health's Task Force on Production and Supply of Vaccines, and in the spring of 1977 she was one of the persons assembled by H.E.W. Secretary Joseph A. Califano (under the chairmanship of Dr. David E. Rogers) to aid in the politically delicate decision concerning the formulation of influenza vaccine for the 1977–1978 season.

ALFRED W. CROSBY, Jr. was born in 1931 in Boston, Massachusetts. He attended public schools in Greater Boston and graduated from Harvard with an A.B. in history in 1952. After three years in the Army, he returned to Massachusetts to do graduate work, receiving an A.M.T. from the Harvard School of Education in 1956 and a Ph.D. in history from Boston University in 1961.

Although neither his formal training nor his early publications suggest any special interest in medical history, he turned to that field in 1967 with the publication of "Conquistador y Pestilencia: The First New World Pandemic and the Fall of the Great Indian Empires" in the *Hispanic American Historical Review* and has been involved in the history of infectious diseases ever since. Greenwood Press has published his two books on the subject, *The Columbian Exchange: Biological and Cultural Consequences of 1492* in 1972 and his most recent, a book on the influenza pandemic of the World War I era, *Epidemic and Peace, 1918,* which won the 1976 American Medical Writers' Association prize as the best volume on a medical subject for laymen.

He is currently a member of the University of Texas at Austin History Department and American Studies Program.

ARTHUR J. VISELTEAR, Ph.D., M.P.H. is an associate professor of public health and research associate in the history of medicine at the Yale University School of Medicine. He received his B.A. degree from Tulane University, and his doctorate in history and master of public health degree from U.C.L.A. At Yale since 1969, he teaches the history of medicine and public health and three seminars which consider "History, Politics, and the Policy of Health." In 1974 he was one of the inaugural group of six Robert Wood Johnson Health Policy Fellows selected for a year of seminar and Congressional assignment in Washington, D.C. As a fellow, and subsequenty as consultant to the Senate Committee on Labor and Public Welfare (1975–1976), he had principal staff responsibility for preventive medicine, health education, and clinical laboratory legislation. Dr. Viseltear is an elected member of the governing council of the American Public Health Association, a former member of the National Institutes of Health Special Study Section on the History of the Life Sciences, adviser to Yale's "Contemporary Medical Care and Health Policy Collection," and has served on the editorial boards of the *Journal of the History of Medicine and Allied Sciences, Medical Care,* and the *Yale Journal of Biology and Medicine.* Dr. Viseltear is author of numerous articles, reports, and chapters which have been published in academic journals, textbooks, and monographs and of two U.S. Senate Reports.

J. DONALD MILLAR, M.D., D.T.P.H., was graduated from the University of Richmond in 1956 and the Medical College of Virginia in 1959. After 2 years as an intern in medical residency at the University of Utah Affiliated Hospitals, he entered the U. S. Public Health Service in 1961 as a field epidemiologist in the Epidemic Intelligence Service of the Center for Disease Control. Since then, as a career officer, he has held various positions at the Center. From 1966 to 1970, he was in charge of the highly successful Smallpox Eradication Program and since 1970 has directed the Bureau of State Services, which comprises the Center's activities in venereal disease control, tuberculosis control, immunization, and environmental health services. He was chosen to direct the Center's participation in the National Influenza Immunization Program of 1976.